MICROANGIOPATHY

Edited by **Raimondo De Cristofaro**

Microangiopathy
Edited by Raimondo De Cristofaro

Published by InTech

Janeza Trdine 9, 51000 Rijeka, Croatia

Publishing Process Manager Romana Vukelic

Technical Editor Teodora Smiljanic

Cover Designer InTech Design Team

Additional hard copies can be obtained from orders@intechopen.com

Microangiopathy, Edited by Raimondo De Cristofaro
p. cm.
ISBN 978-953-51-0419-3

For EU product safety concerns:
IN TECH d.o.o., Prolaz Marije Krucifikse Kozulić 3, 51000 Rijeka, Croatia,
info@intechopen.com or visit our website at intechopen.com.

Meet the editor

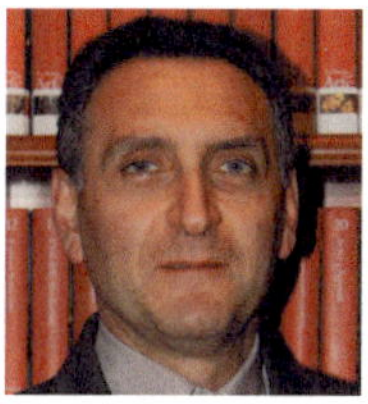

Dr. Raimondo De Cristofaro was born in Naples, Italy, in1960. He obtained his M.D. degree and specialization in Hematology and Internal Medicine at the Catholic UniversitySchool of Medicine of Rome. He worked as Visiting Research Assistant, Dept. of Chemistry and Biochemistry, University of Colorado, Boulder, CO, USA and as Research Associate at the Dept. of Biochemistry and Molecular Biophysics, Washington University, St. Louis, MO, U.S.A. Since 2006 he is Associate Professor of Internal Medicine, at the Catholic University School of Medicine. He is member of several national and international scientific societies in the field of hematology and internal medicine. Dr. De Cristofaro's clinical and research experience concerns diagnosis and treatment of thrombotic diseases and laboratory and clinical evaluation of hemostatic disorders.

Contents

Preface

Microangiopathies are pathological processes causing degenerative disorders of small vessels and involved in a wealth of different diseases. The circulatory problems stemming from microangiopathic disorders may be responsible for failure of individual or multiple organs. Microangiopathies are indeed one of the most common disorders characterized by high morbility and mortality in the affected patients. The knowledge of the mechanisms involved in the genesis of microangiopathies has been strongly expanded in the past few years. Many studies have revealed very complicated processes both at cellular and molecular level. However, much work remains to define the diversity of different pathogenetic mechanisms leading to microangiopathic disorders to provide appropriate prevention and treatment strategies.

This volume contains four informative chapters contributed by experts in their field and provides illustrative examples of relevant mechanisms responsible for different forms of microangiopathies and how this body of evidences can be harnessed to define new strategies of therapeutic intervention.

In Chapter 1, Lancellotti et al. analyze the canonical forms of thrombotic microangiopathies arising from perturbation of the proteolytic processing of von Willebrand factor due to deficiency of ADAMTS13 activity. The main mechanisms of these disorders in the canonical and atypical forms were analyzed and discussed together with old and novel therapeutic strategies used to contrast both the cause and the effects of these diseases.

In Chapter 2 Narimatsu reviews from a pathological and clinical standpoint a particular form of thrombotic microangiopathy that frequently occurs in the intestinal vessels in hematopoietic stem-cell transplantation recipients. In the same chapter Fatih Erbey reviews the transplant-associated thrombotic microangiopathy with emphasis on the clinical and therapeutic aspects concerning pediatric patients.

In chapter 3 Kuang-Yu Jen and Zoltan G. Laszik analyzes the pathologic manifestations and molecular pathologenesis of preeclampsia with a special emphasis on the renal effects of this disease.

Finally, in chapter 4 Vojtková et al. review the ethiopathogenesis of the main microangiopathic complications of diabetes mellitus, that are responsible for retinopathy, nephropathy and neuropathy, which heavily affect the morbility and mortality of this increasingly diffuse disease.

I thank all the authors for their excellent contributions and their efforts to submit updated and outstanding chapters. Expert editorial assistance from Romana Vukelic is gratefully acknowledged, especially because she made possible the timely conclusion of the project and was always a valuable source of valuable suggestions.

Prof. Raimondo De Cristofaro
Department of Internal Medicine and Medical Specialties,
Haemostasis Research Center, Catholic University School of Medicine
Italy

Part 1

Stem Cells Transplantation-Associated Microangiopathies

1

Intestinal Thrombotic Microangiopathy After Hematopoietic Stem Cell Transplantation

Hiroto Narimatsu
Advanced Molecular Epidemiology Research Institute, Faculty of Medicine, Yamagata University, Yamagata, Japan

1. Introduction

Thrombotic microangiopathy (TMA) is a significant complication following hematopoietic stem-cell transplantation (HSCT), which is also described as transplant-associated microangiopathy (TAM). Endothelial injuries from multiple factors contribute to the formation of widespread platelet thrombi within the microvasculature, causing hemolytic anemia and damage to various organs(Daly *et al*, 2002a; Daly *et al*, 2002b; Nishida *et al*, 2004; Pettitt & Clark, 1994; Shimoni *et al*, 2004; Zeigler *et al*, 1996; Zeigler *et al*, 1995). Owing to the difficulty in making a definitive diagnosis of TMA in HSCT recipients, it is usually diagnosed based on clinical and laboratory findings, such as serum lactic dehydrogenase (LD) levels and the percentage of fragmented erythrocytes (Martinez *et al*, 2005; Oran *et al*, 2007; Zeigler *et al*, 1995).

However, these findings are frequently nonspecific, because they are influenced by many other clinical events. Some research group has been reported case series involving TMA with steroid-refractory diarrhea. They showed that TMA frequently involves the gastrointestinal tract in HSCT recipients (Inamoto *et al*, 2009; Narimatsu *et al*, 2005; Nishida *et al*, 2004).

The transplantation-related TMA has different clinical features and outcomes from TMA in the patients with other situations. In this chapter, I describe clinical feature and treatment of the transplantation-related TMA.

2. Classic and intestinal TMA – Clinical manifestations

The most common criteria for classic TMA diagnosis following HSCT are the signs of microangiopathic hemolysis (Martinez *et al*, 2005; Oran *et al*, 2007). On the other hand, in the patients with intestinal TMA, red cell fragmentation and serum LD elevation were usually mild or absent, and serum haptoglobin levels were detectable(Inamoto *et al*, 2009; Narimatsu *et al*, 2005; Nishida *et al*, 2004). Postmortem studies failed to find any evidence of TMA other than in the intestine(Narimatsu *et al*, 2005). Neither renal dysfunction nor neurologic abnormalities were not usually present in those patients. Based on the conventional pentad of HUS/TTP, TMA was not diagnosed in any of them in intestinal TMA. These findings suggest a difference in pathogenesis between intestinal TMA(Inamoto *et al*, 2009; Narimatsu *et al*, 2005; Nishida *et al*, 2004) following HSCT and either classic TTP (Furlan *et al*, 1998) or classic TMA following HSCT(Allford *et al*, 2002; Nishida *et al*, 2004).

The differences in the observations between classic TMA and intestinal TMA can be explained by several reasons, such as the conditioning agents and patients' backgrounds. It may be also explained by following reasons. Clinicians and pathologists might not be commonly aware of TMA and could possibly have misinterpreted it as GVHD or infectious colitis. A pathological diagnosis of TMA can be difficult to make. Thrombolysis, which might occur after death, might have masked the pathological findings of TMA at autopsy (Iwata *et al*, 2001). However, those explanations failed to explain this reason. Thus, further investigation can allow a proper interpretation of the various published reports.

3. Diagnosis of intestinal TMA

Total colonoscopy from the rectum to the terminal ileum with biopsy is required for the diagnosis of intestinal TMA. The patients had focal TMA lesions of various distributions. Thus, biopsy of the rectum alone might have missed the diagnosis of TMA. Colonoscopic findings of TMA were diverse (Narimatsu *et al*, 2005). It was difficult to differentiate TMA from intestinal GVHD (Iqbal *et al*, 2000; Martin *et al*, 2004) and CMV colitis.(Meyers *et al*, 1986) Furthermore, TMA was complicated with GVHD and CMV colitis in many patients (Inamoto *et al*, 2009; Narimatsu *et al*, 2005). Macroscopic observation alone is not sufficient to make a diagnosis of TMA. Laboratory findings alone are also not useful in previous studies (Inamoto *et al*, 2009; Narimatsu *et al*, 2005; Nishida *et al*, 2004). Clinically available risk factors were also not identified in previous studies; laboratory data such as LD at the time of colonoscopy were not significantly different between patients with and without TMA. Thus, a biopsy and a pathological examination extending from the rectum to the terminal ileum are probably necessary to make a definite diagnosis in patients with diarrhea.

4. Pathological features

Suggested mechanisms on onset of intestinal TMA was shown in Figure 1; there is limited information on the pathogenesis of intestinal TMA(Inamoto *et al*, 2009; Narimatsu *et al*, 2005; Nishida *et al*, 2004). Classic TMA after myeloablative HSCT has a multifactorial etiology that includes immunosuppressive agents,(Pham *et al*, 2000; Trimarchi *et al*, 1999) total body irradiation (TBI) (Ballermann, 1998), CMV infection (Takatsuka *et al*, 2003), and acute GVHD (Ertault-Daneshpouy *et al*, 2004). These factors injure the vascular endothelium of many organs (Pettitt & Clark, 1994). In contrast, particular factors specifically affecting the gastrointestinal system are largely involved in the etiology of intestinal TMA after HSCT. It should be noted that most patients with intestinal TMA had overlapping gastrointestinal GVHD and/or CMV colitis(Narimatsu *et al*, 2005). An animal study has demonstrated that the vascular endothelium is a target of alloimmunity (Ertault-Daneshpouy *et al*, 2004). The previous report by us supports this hypothesis(Narimatsu *et al*, 2005). GVHD was associated with gastrointestinal TMA, and the association could partly explain why TMA was located in the gut. It is reasonable to assume that GVHD damages the gastrointestinal endothelium, leading to the development of intestinal TMA. Regimen-related toxicity (RRT) of the gut is known to increase the risk of intestinal GVHD.(Goldberg *et al*, 2005) Gastrointestinal damage due to preparative regimens might contribute to the development of intestinal TMA. In our previous study, CMV infection, which is another putative etiology of TMA,(Takatsuka *et al*, 2003) was documented in 4 patients, and all were located in the gut. (Narimatsu et al, 2005) CMV colitis might be associated with intestinal TMA following HSCT.

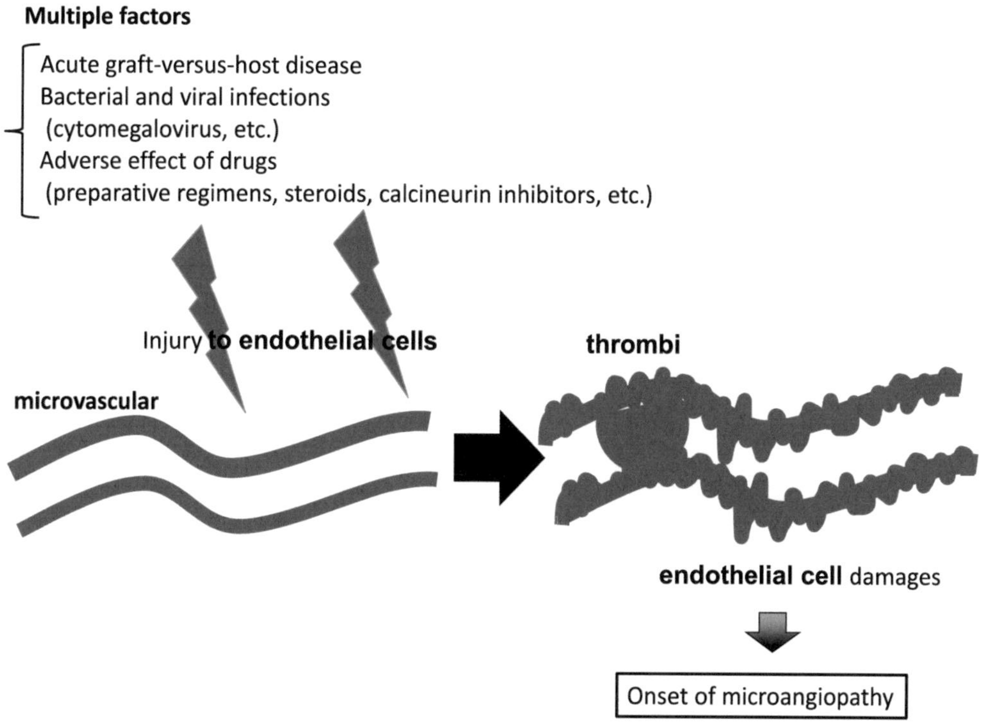

Fig. 1. Suggested mechanisms on onset of intestinal TMA

Inamoto et al presented the usefulness of Immunostainings(Inamoto *et al*, 2009). They made histopathological diagnosis of "intestinal TAM" by the presence of microangiopathy with ischemic (noninflammatory) crypt loss. Microangiopathy was confirmed by hematoxylin-eosin staining and CD34 immunostaining. The clues for endothelial injury are swollen endothelial cells and denuded endothelial cells. Ischemic changes followed by microangiopathy included individual non-inflammatory crypt degeneration with detachment and apoptosis of epithelial cells, wedge-shaped segmental injury and interstitial edema with hemorrhage or fragmented RBCs. Although, pathological definition of intestinal TMA is uncertain, these pathological findings are worth investigating.

5. Treatment

While the appropriate treatment of intestinal TMA is unknown, a published series of cases suggests that reducing the dose of immunosuppressants may be effective for intestinal TMA as well as classic TMA.(Inamoto *et al*, 2009; Nishida *et al*, 2004) On the other hand, our study group suggested that patients with intestinal GVHD and TMA could be improved without immunosuppressant reduction. This observation would indicate that the management of GVHD, rather than immunosuppressant reduction, is important in the treatment of intestinal TMA. In fact, the reduction of immunosuppressants to prevent vascular endothelial damage would aggravate GVHD, and increase the risk of TMA progression. (Narimatsu et al, 2005) Considering these possibilities, one should be vigilant when deciding on the dose of immunosuppressant for TMA after HSCT.

The treatments used for classic TTP, such as fresh frozen plasma and plasma exchange, have been tried for TMA after bone marrow transplantation.(Allford *et al*, 2002) However, the efficacy of these treatments in patients with intestinal TMA remains unclear. Minimizing the damage to the intestinal mucosa and the vascular endothelium would be more desirable for the management of intestinal TMA than the treatments designed for classic TTP.

6. Conclusion and future direction

The intestinal TMA is a significant complication after HSCT. When transplant recipients develop refractory diarrhea, Intestinal TMA needs to be included in the differential diagnoses. However, conventional diagnostic criteria can overlook TMA. Thus, the diagnosis of intestinal TMA after HSCT requires endoscopy with biopsy.

7. References

Allford SL, Bird JM, Marks DI (2002) Thrombotic thrombocytopenic purpura following stem cell transplantation. *Leuk Lymphoma* Vol. 43 No.(10): pp 1921-6,

Ballermann BJ (1998) Endothelial cell activation. *Kidney Int* Vol. 53 No.(6): pp 1810-26,

Daly AS, Hasegawa WS, Lipton JH, Messner HA, Kiss TL (2002a) Transplantation-associated thrombotic microangiopathy is associated with transplantation from unrelated donors, acute graft-versus-host disease and venoocclusive disease of the liver. *Transfus Apher Sci* Vol. 27 No.(1): pp 3-12, 1473-0502 (Print) 1473-0502 (Linking)

Daly AS, Xenocostas A, Lipton JH (2002b) Transplantation-associated thrombotic microangiopathy: twenty-two years later. *Bone Marrow Transplant* Vol. 30 No.(11): pp 709-15, 0268-3369 (Print) 0268-3369 (Linking)

Ertault-Daneshpouy M, Leboeuf C, Lemann M, Bouhidel F, Ades L, Gluckman E, Socie G, Janin A (2004) Pericapillary hemorrhage as criterion of severe human digestive graft-versus-host disease. *Blood* Vol. 103 No.(12): pp 4681-4,

Furlan M, Robles R, Galbusera M, Remuzzi G, Kyrle PA, Brenner B, Krause M, Scharrer I, Aumann V, Mittler U, Solenthaler M, Lammle B (1998) von Willebrand Factor-Cleaving Protease in Thrombotic Thrombocytopenic Purpura and the Hemolytic-Uremic Syndrome. *N Engl J Med* Vol. 339 No.(22): pp 1578-1584,

Goldberg J, Jacobsohn DA, Zahurak ML, Vogelsang GB (2005) Gastrointestinal toxicity from the preparative regimen is associated with an increased risk of graft-versus-host disease. *Biol Blood Marrow Transplant* Vol. 11 No.(2): pp 101-7,

Inamoto Y, Ito M, Suzuki R, Nishida T, Iida H, Kohno A, Sawa M, Murata M, Nishiwaki S, Oba T, Yanada M, Naoe T, Ichihashi R, Fujino M, Yamaguchi T, Morishita Y, Hirabayashi N, Kodera Y, Miyamura K (2009) Clinicopathological manifestations and treatment of intestinal transplant-associated microangiopathy. *Bone Marrow Transplant* Vol. 44 No.(1): pp 43-9, 1476-5365 (Electronic) 0268-3369 (Linking)

Iqbal N, Salzman D, Lazenby AJ, Wilcox CM (2000) Diagnosis of gastrointestinal graft-versus-host disease. *Am J Gastroenterol* Vol. 95 No.(11): pp 3034-8,

Iwata H, Kami M, Hori A, Hamaki T, Takeuchi K, Mutou Y (2001) An autopsy-based retrospective study of secondary thrombotic thrombocytopenic purpura. *Haematologica* Vol. 86 No.(6): pp 669-70,

Martin PJ, McDonald GB, Sanders JE, Anasetti C, Appelbaum FR, Deeg HJ, Nash RA, Petersdorf EW, Hansen JA, Storb R (2004) Increasingly frequent diagnosis of acute gastrointestinal graft-versus-host disease after allogeneic hematopoietic cell transplantation. *Biol Blood Marrow Transplant* Vol. 10 No.(5): pp 320-7,

Martinez MT, Bucher C, Stussi G, Heim D, Buser A, Tsakiris DA, Tichelli A, Gratwohl A, Passweg JR (2005) Transplant-associated microangiopathy (TAM) in recipients of allogeneic hematopoietic stem cell transplants. *Bone Marrow Transplant* Vol. 36 No.(11): pp 993-1000, 0268-3369 (Print) 0268-3369 (Linking)

Meyers JD, Flournoy N, Thomas ED (1986) Risk factors for cytomegalovirus infection after human marrow transplantation. *J Infect Dis* Vol. 153 No.(3): pp 478-88,

Narimatsu H, Kami M, Hara S, Matsumura T, Miyakoshi S, Kusumi E, Kakugawa Y, Kishi Y, Murashige N, Yuji K, Masuoka K, Yoneyama A, Wake A, Morinaga S, Kanda Y, Taniguchi S (2005) Intestinal thrombotic microangiopathy following reduced-intensity umbilical cord blood transplantation. *Bone Marrow Transplant* Vol. 36: pp 517-23,

Nishida T, Hamaguchi M, Hirabayashi N, Haneda M, Terakura S, Atsuta Y, Imagama S, Kanie T, Murata M, Taji H, Suzuki R, Morishita Y, Kodera Y (2004) Intestinal thrombotic microangiopathy after allogeneic bone marrow transplantation: a clinical imitator of acute enteric graft-versus-host disease. *Bone Marrow Transplant* Vol. 33 No.(11): pp 1143-50, 0268-3369 (Print) 0268-3369 (Linking)

Oran B, Donato M, Aleman A, Hosing C, Korbling M, Detry MA, Wei C, Anderlini P, Popat U, Shpall E, Giralt S, Champlin RE (2007) Transplant-associated microangiopathy in patients receiving tacrolimus following allogeneic stem cell transplantation: risk factors and response to treatment. *Biology of blood and marrow transplantation : journal of the American Society for Blood and Marrow Transplantation* Vol. 13 No.(4): pp 469-77, 1083-8791 (Print) 1083-8791 (Linking)

Pettitt AR, Clark RE (1994) Thrombotic microangiopathy following bone marrow transplantation. *Bone Marrow Transplant* Vol. 14 No.(4): pp 495-504, 0268-3369 (Print) 0268-3369 (Linking)

Pham PT, Peng A, Wilkinson AH, Gritsch HA, Lassman C, Pham PC, Danovitch GM (2000) Cyclosporine and tacrolimus-associated thrombotic microangiopathy. *Am J Kidney Dis* Vol. 36 No.(4): pp 844-50,

Shimoni A, Yeshurun M, Hardan I, Avigdor A, Ben-Bassat I, Nagler A (2004) Thrombotic microangiopathy after allogeneic stem cell transplantation in the era of reduced-intensity conditioning: The incidence is not reduced. *Biology of blood and marrow transplantation : journal of the American Society for Blood and Marrow Transplantation* Vol. 10 No.(7): pp 484-93, 1083-8791 (Print) 1083-8791 (Linking)

Takatsuka H, Wakae T, Mori A, Okada M, Fujimori Y, Takemoto Y, Okamoto T, Kanamaru A, Kakishita E (2003) Endothelial damage caused by cytomegalovirus and human herpesvirus-6. *Bone Marrow Transplant* Vol. 31 No.(6): pp 475-9,

Trimarchi HM, Truong LD, Brennan S, Gonzalez JM, Suki WN (1999) FK506-associated thrombotic microangiopathy: report of two cases and review of the literature. *Transplantation* Vol. 67 No.(4): pp 539-44,

Zeigler ZR, Rosenfeld CS, Andrews DF, 3rd, Nemunaitis J, Raymond JM, Shadduck RK, Kramer RE, Gryn JF, Rintels PB, Besa EC, George JN (1996) Plasma von Willebrand Factor Antigen (vWF:AG) and thrombomodulin (TM) levels in Adult Thrombotic Thrombocytopenic Purpura/Hemolytic Uremic Syndromes (TTP/HUS) and bone marrow transplant-associated thrombotic microangiopathy (BMT-TM). *Am J Hematol* Vol. 53 No.(4): pp 213-20, 0361-8609 (Print)0361-8609 (Linking)

Zeigler ZR, Shadduck RK, Nemunaitis J, Andrews DF, Rosenfeld CS (1995) Bone marrow transplant-associated thrombotic microangiopathy: a case series. *Bone Marrow Transplant* Vol. 15 No.(2): pp 247-53, 0268-3369 (Print)0268-3369 (Linking)

2

Transplant-Associated Thrombotic Microangiopathy in Childhood

Fatih Erbey
Medicalpark Bahcelievler Hospital, Department of Pediatric Hematology/Oncology & Pediatric BMT Unit, Istanbul, Turkey

1. Introduction

Transplant-associated thrombotic microangiopathy (TMA) among early complications after hematopoietic stem cell transplantation (HSCT) in children was first described in 1980 (1). Incidence varies between centers with an average of 7.9% (0.5-63.6%) (2-4).

Vascular endothelium is damaged by toxic agents during the preparation regimen for stem cell transplantation. Microthrombi develop in small arterioles and capillaries and cause partial obstruction. Erithrocytes are subjected to mechanical trauma, and as a result, to hemolysis and fragmentation. Patients have clinical symptoms similar to thrombotic thrombocytopenic purpura (TTP) and Hemolytic Uremic Syndrome (HUS).

2. Pathology

TMA is a pathological definition and characterized by fibrinoid necrosis in vessel walls and arteriolar thrombus (5). Following intravascular thrombocyte activation due to microscopic damage, thrombus rich in thrombocytes develops in microcirculation. This process depletes thrombocytes. On the other hand, blood cells are mechanically damaged due to microcirculation obstructed by fibrin particles or microthrombus. The clinical picture is microangiopathic hemolytic anemia and thrombocytopenia.

3. Pathogenesis

TMA has the characteristics of TTP and HUS. It is seen not only in HSCT but also in all patients who had chemotherapy or radiotherapy, in systemic sclerosis, systemic lupus erythematosus, antiphospholipid syndrome, malign hypertension, preeclampsia-eclampsia, infections, cancers, renal transplantation and with drugs (5-8).

In primary TTP, there is a deficiency of metalloproteinases which adhere to the very large Von Willebrand factor (UL vWF) multimers in vivo and sweep them away from the endothelial cells (8-10). This protease is called as "ADAMTS13" and belongs to a disintegrin and metalloproteinase with thrombospondin type 1 repeats family (11-15). Severe ADAMTS13 deficiency (activity <5%) is seen in 33-100% of patients with primary TTP (16). Consequently, newly formed autoantibodies in primary TTP inhibit ADAMTS13 and thus the unswept vWF multimers and thrombocytes aggregate causing a thrombocyte-rich-thrombus formation in microvascular bed. ADAMTS13 deficiency is found rarely in TMA associated with other causes excluding TTP (4).

While the pathogenesis in transplant-associated TMA is not very clear, it is believed that the disease process starts with endothelial damage. In this case, the abnormalities in vascular endothelium are independent from ADAMTS13 deficiency. Laurence et al (17), showed that apoptosis in microvascular endothelial cells can be induced by plasma from patients with primer TTP and HUS in vitro (18). They also demonstrated enhanced apoptosis of microvascular endothelial cells in vivo in patient with TTP (19). These studies revealed induction of Fas (CD95) in endothelial cells after exposure to TTP plasma, which results in apoptosis of human cells (17-19). On the basis of their findings, they proposed that induction of endothelial cell injury was an important component of the pathogenesis of TMA. This form of injury has been shown to correlate with the generation of platelet microparticles in vitro and in patients with classical TTP (20). The mechanism of apoptosis appears to be linked to the rapid induction of Fas (CD95) on cultured microvascular endothelium and can be blocked in vitro by anti-Fas antibodies, normal cryo-poor plasma and low concentrations of the nonspecific protease and endonuclease inhibitor aurintricarboxylic acid. Inhibitors of caspases-1 and 3 and overexpression of Bcl-X_L in cultured microvascular endothelial cells suppress the induction of apoptosis in these cells by TTP plasma (21). Apoptosis of microvascular endothelial cells may represent a final common pathway of injury leading to the clinical expression of microangiopathic hemolytic anemia.

Endothelial damage causes the secretion of thrombocyte aggregating agent to the microvascular circulation. There is an increase in thrombomodulin, P-selectin (GMP-140) and tissue plasminogen activator levels (22). Causes of endothelial damage include cyclophosphamide, nitrosureas (busulfan), chemotherapeutics, such as platin based agents, radiotherapy, cyclosporine and tacrolimus for greft versus host disease (GVHD) prophylaxis, cytokines secreted in acute GVHD and infections (fungal, CMV, HHV-6) (Figure 1) (23,24).

The development of the scenario after 3-6 months following chemotherapy/ radiotherapy suggests that direct antibodies are formed against the endothelium and thrombocyte glycoprotein IV (CD 36) or other intracellular endothelial antigenic targets. IL-1, IL-6, soluble IL-2 receptor and TNFα plasma levels are increased in primary TTP. The histopathologic determinant for TTP/HUS is the presence of intravascular thrombocyte aggregating agents with abundant vWF content as seen in disseminated intravascular coagulation (DIC) [without soluble coagulation factor activation (eg. fibrin deposition)]. There's abnormal vWF profile in plasma of the patients with primary and transplant-associated disease. The affinity of vWF multimers to bind thrombocytes is high. Specifically, in arteriolar vessels where the flow is high, the aggregated thrombocytes form nidus onto which the ULvWF multimers cling. Cryoprecipitate with reduced plasma causes less thrombocyte aggregation activity by reducing the ULvWF. Due to this reductase activity, blood exchange using cryoprecipitate with reduced plasma is performed in severe TTP/HUS (23-25). In addition, thrombomodulin which is related to endothelial cell damage, plasminogen activator inhibitor-1 and soluble intercellular adhesion molecule increase in patients' serum (26-31). Increased levels of IL-1, IL-8, TNFα and IFNγ expand the inflammation mediated tissue damage via direct toxicity to endothelium. This may lead to acute GVHD or hepatic veno-occlusive disease (VOD) (32-36). Some investigators even think that the transplant-associated TMA is an endothelial form of GVHD (37).

Cyclosporine when used in GVHD prophylaxis, increases the thromboxane A_2 production and decreases the prostaglandin I_2 production (38, 39). Cyclosporine and most probably tacrolimus show direct toxicity to endothelium (40-45) and addition of sirolimus to calcinorin inhibitors potentializes these toxic effects (46-48).

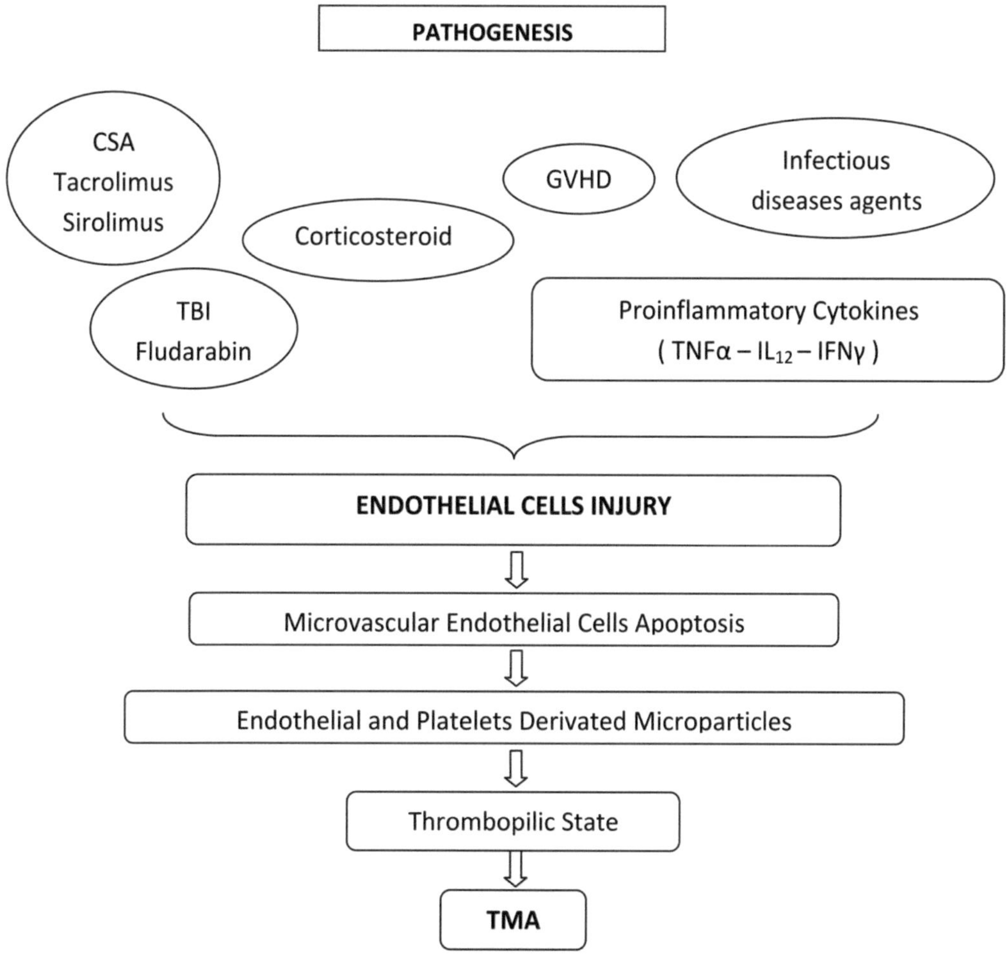

Endothelial cell injury and apoptosis have been associated with generation of endothelial microparticles that may be relaased in to the circulation. Release of endothelial microparticles has been associated with procoagulant activity. Furthermore, endothelial microparticles induce platelet aggregation, and thus by inducing microthrombosis could predispose to TMA.

Abreviations: CSA; cyclosporin-A, GVHD; Graft-versus-host disease, TBI; Total body irradiation, TMA; thrombotic microangiopathy

Fig. 1. Pathogenesis of Transplantation associated thrombotic microangiopathy.

4. Risk factors for TMA

1. Female gender
2. Age: less frequent in children compared to adults.
3. Donor type: more frequent in unrelated donors and mismatch related donors.
4. Severity of the primary disease.
5. Nonmyeloablative transplant (Fludarabine based conditioning regimens)
6. High dose busulfan use (16 mg/kg)
7. Use of antithymocyte globulin or total body irradiation
8. Presence of 2nd or more degree acute GVHD
9. Cyclosporine, tacrolimus, sirolimus use
10. Neuroblastoma patients specifically with a history of cisplatin treatment
11. Presence of an infection, especially CMV. We reported that in a patient who developed TMA together with CMV infection, TMA signs resolved completely after successful treatment of CMV infection (49).
12. Stem cell source; Elliott et al. (12) reported that 4 of the 25 (16 %) bone morrow transplantations from a HLA full matched sibling resulted in TMA, however, none of the 45 peripheral stem cell transplantations from a HLA full matched sibling resulted in TMA. They defined the use of bone marrow as a stem cell source as a risk factor. They also stated that prospective, large and comparative studies were needed in order to understand the relationship between TMA and the stem cell source. As opposed to their results, 3 of the 18 patients (16.6. %) in our study who used peripheral blood for the source of stem cells developed TMA while none of the 32 patients who used the bone morrow developed it. We concluded that the use of the peripheral stem cell was a risk factor for TMA (50). Like Elliott et al., we also think that prospective, large and comparative studies are needed in order to understand the relationship between TMA and the stem cell source.

5. Clinical signs

Signs develop in an average of 44-171 days after the transplantation. In 2/3 of the cases, the disease occurs before 100 days (51). Erythrocytes are fragmented by microangiopathic damage and erythrocyte turnover increases without immune mediated hemolysis or DIC. Peripheral smear shows fragmented erythrocytes (schistocytes). Mild hemolysis, severe anemia, thrombocytopenia, fever, hematuria, mental disability, and kidney failure requiring dialysis may be present in patients. Biochemically, serum lactate dehydrogenase (LDH) is increased, haptoglobulin level is decreased. In addition, indirect hyperbilirubinemia and hemoglobinuria may be seen.

Fragmented erythrocyte ratio is 4-10% in transplant-associated TMA. Nucleated erythrocytes may be found in peripheral circulation. Thrombocyte consumption is increased although DIC is not present. Plasma vWF level is high albeit not pathognomonic. Studies demonstrate that vWF level increases more in allogeneic stem cell recipients compared to autologus recipients. The highest levels of vWF are seen in 3-4 months after the transplantation when TMA is also clinically presented.

6. Diagnostic criteria for transplant-associated TMA

In a study by George et al (2), a total of 28 parameters were detected to be used for diagnosis in various centers. It is also observed that such a wide range of diagnostic criteria use caused variability in incidence ranging from 0.5-63.6%. As a result, an international research group was organized and a consensus on diagnostic criteria was reached. According to this consensus, the following diagnostic criteria were determined (3).

1. Presence of schistocytes
2. Presence of prolonged or progressive thrombocytopenia (<50x10^9/l) or 50% or more decrease in the previous thrombocyte count)
3. Sudden and persistent LDH increase
4. Decrease in hemoglobin concentration or increase in transfusion needs
5. Decrease in serum haptoglobulin level

Each criteria needs to be fulfilled for diagnosis. Sensitivity and specificity are 80% (3).

7. Differential diagnosis

7.1 Cyclosporine toxicity

Isolated microangiopathy: 1-2% erythrocyte fragmentation is seen in most patients treated with cyclosporine or tacrolimus after transplantation. At toxic serum levels of these drugs, fragmented erythrocytes increase to 3-4%, indirect bilirubin is increased and reticulocytosis is observed.When cyclosporine dose is decreased and the serum drug levels turn to therapeutic levels, hemolysis and renal effects return to normal. Vitamin E may treat hemolysis after transplantation.

Cyclosporine associated central nervous system dysfunction: This picture is frequently mistaken as TMA in the first 6 months after transplantation. Seizures, alterations in conciousness, apraxia/ataxia or cortical blindness may be seen in patients. These symptoms are usually related with uncontrolled hypertension, renal tubular acidosis and magnesium loss. Symptoms resolve within 48-72 hours with the reduction of cyclosporine dose. In treatment, cyclosporine should be stopped temporarily, another drug should be used for GVHD prophylaxis, hypertension should be controlled, magnesium should be replaced and if necessary an antiepileptic drugs should be used. If cyclosporine is restarted in patients with cortical blindness, speech disturbance or coma, symptoms may reappear. In some patients cyclosporine maybe replaced by tacrolimus uneventfully. Behavioural disturbances, alterations in conciousness level and seizures are observed both in cyclosporine toxicity and TMA. Cortical blindness and apraxia/ataxia are more frequently associated with cyclosporine toxicity and are reversible (23).

7.2 Immune hemolytic anemia

Immune hemolytic anemia may develop after transplantation, especially in patients who had received multiple transfussions prior to HSCT (eg patients with hemoglobinopathies). There is increased need for erythrocyte supplementation in these patients. Fragmented erythrocytes are detected in peripheral smear, reticulocyte count, LDH and indirect bilirubin levels are increased, haptoglobulin is decreased. While direct antiglobulin (direct coombs) test is positive in these patients, it is negative in transplant-associated TMA.

7.3 Disseminated intravascular coagulation

Hemostatic system is a dynamic system that under normal conditions is balanced by thrombus formation via the conversion of prothrombin to thrombin and thrombus degradation via elimination of trombin with antithrombin before it promotes coagulation. Disturbance of this balance by any reason leads to aggregation of fibrin and thrombin and thus, to this clinical condition secondary to the activation of fibrinolysis which may result in death. Fibrin is widely accumulated (microthrombus) in small vessels of various organs due to thrombin effect. Fibrin accumulation leads to consumption of mainly thrombocytes and fibrinogen, several coagulation factors (II, V, VIII) and erythrocytes. Accumulated fibrin in vessels is lysed when the fibrinolytic system is activated and fibrin degradation products (FDP) pass to the circulation (secondary fibrinolysis). Fibrin aggregates in small vessels may cause ischemic tissue necrosis (bilateral renal necrosis, surrenal necrosis) and in some instances where fibrin ligaments have accumulated to completely obstruct the vessel lumen, microangiopathic hemolytic anemia may develop.

Clinical presentation may vary from being asymptomatic to shock. Bleeding occurs as a result of coagulation factors and platelet depletion. It maybe observed as petechiae and echymosis, oozing from injection sites and gums, subcutaneous hematomas, nasal bleeding, hematuria, gastrointestinal and intracranial hemorrhage.

Ischemic organ damage due to intravascular thrombosis may be seen. Furthermore, in chronic DIC, due to fibrin deposition in glomerules, renal insufficiency characterized by oliguria frequently accompanies the case.

Thrombi and fibrin materials formed as a result of the damage that erythrocytes have incurred during their flow through the vessels, block the vessel lumen. This condition causes microangiopathic hemolytic anemia.

In the diagnosis of DIC; fibrinogen level is low, prothrombin time is prolonged, actiavted partial thromboplastin time is prolonged, factor II, V, VIII and XIII levels are low and thrombocytopenia is present. Final diagnosis is made by the demonstration of fibrinogen-fibrin degradation products in serum using immunoassay. FDP has high levels and fibrin monomer polymerization is prolonged. The D-dimer test is specific for fibrin proteolysis. Fibrin complexes are high in circulation. If the fibrinogen is lower than 1 g/L, thrombin time is prolonged, however if fibrinogen level is higher than 1 g/L and thrombin time is prolonged, this means the FDP is increased.

When microangiopathic hemolytic anemia develops, fragmented erythrocytes are found in peripheral blood smear. Reticulocyte count is increased secondary to hemolysis. Thrombocytopenia and absence of thrombocyte aggregates in peripheral smear may be seen as a result of platelet consumption in microvascular thrombosis and platelet activation of circulating thrombin. Antithrombin III is decreased, euglobulin lysis time is shortened. Search for fibrin monomer formation and fibrinopeptide measurements are more complicated tests however used rarely for confirmation of diagnosis.

8. Treatment

Currently there is no any consensus on the therapy of TMA. However, there is no any randomized trials regarding to treatment. Once transplant-associated TMA is suspected, the potentially blamed drugs such as cyclosporine, tacrolimus or sirolimus should be seized. Necessary immunosupression should be provided by corticosteroid, mycophenolate and azathiopurine. In a patient using cyclosporine, the drug may be replaced by tacrolimus but this usually does not help (52).

8.1 Plasma exchange

Despite limited data, many centers use plasma exchange as part of the treatment in transplant-associated TMA. Plasma exchange using cryoprecipitate with reduced plasma or fresh frozen plasma may be used alone or in combination with staphylococcal protein immunoabsorption. Its efficiency is controversial. Response rate to plasma exchange, when compared with primary TTP (75%), is significantly less in transplant-associated TMA (<50%) (32, 53). Furthermore, the mortality in transplant-associated TMA is greater than 80% when plasma exchange used whereas it is 20% in idiopathic TTP (16, 32, 53-55). Limited response to plasma exchange and high mortality rate despite plasma exchange are associated with ADAMTS13 levels. In primary TTP, ADAMTS13 activity is inhibited by autoantibodies is restored by plasma exchange, thus the underlying disease mechanism is reversed and clinical outcome is positive. However, in transplant-associated TMA, since the case is independent from ADAMTS13 activity the response rates are low in spite of plasma exchange. On the other hand, 28% of patients treated with plasma exchange had complications such as infections due to plasmapheresis catheter or transfused plasma, thrombosis, hemorrhage, pneumothorax, pericardial tamponade, hypoxia, hypotension, serum sickness, and anaphylaxis (56-58).

Based on the absence of convincing data in published series and high complication rates, some researchers emphasize not to use plasma exchange routinely for transplant-associated TMA until new clinical study results are available or at least to rule out other factors that could cause TMA (eg.infections, GVHD) before use (54, 59).

8.2 Defibrotide

Recently, the most pronounced agent is defibrotide, a polideoxyribonucleotide salt. Defibrotide has antithrombotic and thrombolytic activity and inhibits the TNFα mediated endothelial cell apoptosis in-vitro (60). Defibrotide's main effect is local on vascular bed. It does not have a significant effect on systemic coagulation. Defibrotide has protective effects on damaged or activated endothelial cells especially in small vessels. Defibrotide once bound to vascular endothelial cells decreases their procoagulant activity and increases their fibrinolytic potentials. The drug also has anti-inflammatory and anti-ischemic effects (35, 61). The effectivity of defibrotide has been shown in hepatic VOD treatment (35-36). In a study by Corti et al, 12 TMA patients were reported to be treated with defibrotide, 6 patients had complete remission, 3 had partial remission (61). In coclusion, considering the similarity between VOD and transplant-associated TMA and that the endothelial damage is held mainly responsible for pathogenesis, large scale randomized studies with defibrotide are required.

8.3 Other therapeutic approaches

Literature reveals a few other treatment approaches with different outcomes (Table 1). Wollf et al, described complete remission in 9 out of 13 patients with TMA and GVHD whose treatments for GVHD by calcinorin inhibitors were stopped and replaced with anti-CD25 antibody (daclizumab). Five of those patients with complete remission for TMA also had complete remission for GVHD. While 4 patients were still alive 266 days after the transplantation, 1 died due to relapse of the primary disease and the rest 8 died due to infections, GVHD or multiorgan dysfunction (62).

Au et al, treated 5 patients refractory to plasma exchange and high dose corticosteroid therapy with a total of 4 doses of rituximab once a week. Four patients had complete remission, one of which later died due to sepsis. The patient without remission died 3 weeks later due to multiorgan failure (63). The mechanism of action for rituximab in transplant-associated TMA is not clear, nevertheless, is thought to be related with the immunomodulator effectivity of the drug.

Takatsuka et al, used eicasopentaneoic acid (EPA) to decrease the inflammation related complication such as TMA in peritransplantation period. Sixteen patients were enrolled in this study. EPA was started 3 weeks prior to the transplantation in 7 patients who have undergone allogeneic transplantation from unrelated donors and continued up to 180 days after the procedure. EPA was not given to the other 9 patients. All patients had similar preparation regimes and GVHD prophylaxis. Four patients developed TMA and 5 patients died in the group not receiving EPA. In the group receiving EPA, non developed TMA and all survived until 143 days after the transplantation (64).

Kajiume et al used transdermal isosorbide successfully in a case and have not reported any side effects (65).

8.4 Future approaches

TNFα inhibitors such as etanercept and infliximab are demonstrated to be effective in acute GVHD treatment. Theoretically they are thought to be effective in transplant-associated TMA as well (66-71). However, TNFα inhibitors' potentially increasing the risk of opportunistic infections such as fungal and viral infections limits their use (67-70).

Statins decrease the endothelial inflammatory response and myocardial ischemia (72-75). Iloprost is a prostacycline analogue decreasing the endothelial cell damage and the markers increasing during its activation (76). Endothelin receptor antagonists reverse the microvascular damage induced by cyclosporine in vitro (77), shows protective effect against endothelial damage due to ischemia/reperfusion in vivo (78). Edaravone is a free radical scavenger inhibiting the vascular endothelial cell damage in patients with myocardial ischemia and cerebrovascular trauma. In animal models, it decreases the thrombogenesis associated with damaged endothelium via increasing the nitric oxide synthesis (79). Also in animal models, edaravone was found to decrease cysplatin induced renal toxicity (80). Currently edaravone is approved for ischemic stroke treatment only. Table 2 shows agents that have not been used for transplant-associated TMA but have a certain potential to be used.

9. Prognosis

Being a feared complication of HSCT, transplant-associated TMA has bad prognosis. Literature search yields a mortality rate of more than 60% (2). High mortality rate is multifactorial; related not only with TMA associated kidney failure, myocardial dysfunction and brain ischemia but also with other confounding severe complications of transplantation (eg. infections, GVHD). In several series, prognostic factors were evaluated and bad prognostic criteria were listed below (37, 46, 81, 82).

1. Age equal to or greater than 18.
2. Unrelated or haploidentic donor
3. Increased TMA index (LDH/platelet ratio)
4. Schistocyte count > 5-10 hpf
5. Patients not exposed to sirolimus
6. Presence of nephropathy

Additionally, some authors think that delays in diagnosis and/or treatment are also associated with high mortality.

In conclusion, TMA is a severe complication yet to be investigated thoroughly since the pathogenesis is not clear, there is no consensus on treatment and morbidity-mortality rates are high.

10. References

[1] Powles RL, Clink HM, Spence D, Morgenstern G, Watson JG, Selby HJ, et al. Cyclosporine A to prevent graft-versus-host disease in man after allogeneic bone marrow transplantation. Lancet 1980;1:327-9.

[2] George JN, Li X, McMinn JR, Terrell DR, Vesely SK, Selby GB. Thrombotic thrombocytopenic purpura - hemolytic uremic syndrome following allogeneic HPC transplantation: a diagnostic dilemma. Transfusion 2004;44:294-304.

[3] Ruutu T, Barosi G, Benjamin RJ, Clark RE, George JN, Grathwohl A, et al. Diagnostic criteria for hematopoietic stem cell transplant-associated microangiopathy: results of a consensus process by an International Working Group. Haematologica 2007;92:95-100.

[4] Batts ED, Lazarus HM. Diagnosis and treatment of transplantation-associated thrombotic microangiopathy: real progress ora re we waiting? Bone Marrow Transplant 2007;40:709-19.

[5] Laszik Z, Silva F. Hemolytic-uremic syndrome, thrombotic thrombocytopenic purpura, and systemic sclerosis (systemic scleroderma). In: Jennet JC, Olson JL, Schwartz MM, Silva FG (eds). Heptinstall's Pathology of the Kidney. Lippincott-Raven: Philadelphia, 1998, 1003–57.

[6] Sadler JE, Poncz M. Antibody-mediated thrombotic disorders: idiopathic thrombotic thrombocytopenic purpura and heparin-induced thrombocytopenia. In: Lichtman MA, Beutler E, Kipps TJ, Seligsohn U, Kaushansky K, Prchal J (eds). Williams Hematology. McGraw-Hill: New York, 2006, 2031–54.

[7] Arslan Ş. Hemolitik üremik sendromlar. T Klin Pediatri Özel 2004; 2:104-11.

[8] Çelik A. Trombotik trombositopenik purpura ve Hemolitik üremik sendrom. T Klinikleri J Int Med Sci 2007; 3(4):30-35.

[9] Furlan M, Robles R, Solenthaler M, Wassmer M, Sandoz P, Lammle B. Deficient activity of von Willebrand factorcleaving protease in chronic relapsing thrombotic thrombocytopenic purpura. Blood 1997;89:3097–103.

[10] Furlan M, Robles R, Galbusera M, Remuzzi G, Kyrle PA, Brenner B, et al. Von Willebrand factor-cleaving protease in thrombotic thrombocytopenic purpura and the hemolyticuremic syndrome. New Engl J Med 1998;339:1578–84.

[11] Gerritsen HE, Robles R, Lammle B, Furlan M. Partial amino acid sequence of purified von Willebrand factor-cleaving protease. Blood 2001;98:1654–61.

[12] Fujikawa K, Suzuki H, McMullen B, Chung D. Purification of human von Willebrand factor-cleaving protease and its identification as a new member of the metalloproteinase family. Blood 2001;98:1662–66.
[13] Levy GG, Nichols WC, Lian EC, Foroud T, McClintock JN, McGee BM, et al. Mutations in a member of the ADAMTS gene family cause thrombotic thrombocytopenic purpura. Nature 2001;413:488–94.
[14] Soejima K, Mimura N, Hirashima M, Maeda H, Hamamoto T, Nakagaki T, et al. A novel human metalloprotease synthesized in the liver and secreted into the blood: possibly, the von Willebrand factor-cleaving protease? J Biochem (Tokyo) 2001;130:475–80.
[15] Zheng X, Chung D, Takayama TK, Majerus EM, Sadler JE, Fujikawa K. Structure of von Willebrand factor-cleaving protease (ADAMTS13), a metalloprotease involved in thrombotic thrombocytopenic purpura. J Biol Chem 2001;276:41059–63.
[16] Sadler JE. Thrombotic thrombocytopenic purpura: a moving target. Hematology (Am Soc Hematol Educ Program) 2006, 415–20.
[17] Laurence J, Mitra D, Steiner M, Staiano-Coico L, Jaffe E. Plasma from patients with idiopathic and human immunodeficiency virus-associated thrombotic thrombocytopenic purpura induces apoptosis in microvascular endothelial. Blood 1996;87:3245-54.
[18] Mitra D, Jaffe E, Weksler B, Hajjar KA, Soderland C, Laurence J. Thrombotic thrombocytopenic purpura and sporadic hemolytic-uremic syndrome plasmas induced apoptosis in restricted lineages of human microvascular endothelial cells. Blood 1997;89:1224-34.
[19] Dang CT, Magid M, Weksler B, Chadburn A, Laurence J. Enhanced endothelial apoptosis in splenic tissue of patients with thrombotic thrombocytopenic purpura. Blood 1999;93:1264-70.
[20] Jimenez JJ, Jy W, Mauro L, Horstman LL, Ahn YS. Elevated endothelial microparticles in thrombotic thrombocytopenic purpura: findings from brain and renal microvascular cell culture and patients with active disease. Br J Haematol 2001;112:81-90.
[21] Mitra D, Kim J, MacLow C, Karsan A, Laurence J. Role of caspases 1 and 3 and Bcl-2-related molecules in endothelial cell apoptosis associated with thrombotic microangiopathies. Am J Hematol 1998;59:279-87.
[22] Valilis PN, Zeigler ZR, Shadduck RK. A prospective study of bone marrow transplant-associated thrombotic microanjopathy (BMT-TM) in autologous (Auto) and allogeneic (Allo) BMT. Blood 1995;86:970a (abstract).
[23] Sniecinski IJ, O'Donnel MR. Hemolytic complications of hematopoietic cell transplantation. In: Thomas ED, Blume KG, Forman SJ (eds). Hematopoietic cell transplantation 2nd ed. Blackwell Science, USA, 1999, 674-84.
[24] Juckett M, Perry EH, Daniels BS, Weisdorf DJ. Hemolytic uremic syndrome following bone marrow transplantation. Bone Marrow Transplant. 1991;7:405-9.
[25] Moake JL. Studies in the pathophysiology of thrombotic thrombocytopenic purpura. Semin Hematol. 1997;34:83-9.
[26] Testa S, Manna A, Porcellini A, Maffi F, Morstabilini G, Denti N, et al. Increased plasma level of vascular endothelial glycoprotein thrombomodulin as an early indicator of

endothelial damage in bone marrow transplantation. Bone Marrow Transplant 1996;18:383–8.

[27] Richard S, Seigneur M, Blann A, Adams R, Renard M, Puntous M, et al. Vascular endothelial lesion in patients undergoing bone marrow transplantation. Bone Marrow Transplant 1996;18:955–9.

[28] Salat C, Holler E, Kolb HJ, Pihusch R, Reinhardt B, Hiller E. Endothelial cell markers in bone marrow transplant recipients with and without acute graft versus host disease. Bone Marrow Transplant 1997;19:909–14.

[29] Nurnberger W, Michelmann I, Burdach S, Gobel U. Endothelial dysfunction after bone marrow transplantation: increase of soluble thrombomodulin and PAI-1 in patients with multiple transplant-related complications. Ann Hematol 1998;76:61–5.

[30] Kanamori H, Maruta A, Sasaki S, Yamazaki E, Ueda S, Katoh K, et al. Diagnostic value of hemostatic parameters in bone marrow transplant-associated thrombotic microangiopathy. Bone Marrow Transplant 1998;21:705–9.

[31] Takatsuka H, Wakae T, Mori A, Okada M, Fujimori Y, Takemoto Y, et al. Endothelial damage caused by cytomegalovirus and human herpesvirus-6. Bone Marrow Transplant 2003;31:475–9.

[32] Daly AS, Xenocostas A, Lipton JH. Transplantation associated thrombotic microangiopathy: twenty-two years later. Bone Marrow Transplant 2002;30:709-15.

[33] Takatsuka H, Wakae T, Mori A, Okada M, Suehiro A, Okamoto T, et al. Thrombotic thrombocytopenic purpura and hemolytic uremic syndrome following allogeneic bone marrow transplantation. Bone Marrow Transplant 2002;29:907–11.

[34] Qu L, Kiss JE. Thrombotic microangiopathy in transplantation and malignancy. Semin Thromb Hemost 2005;31:691–9.

[35] Richardson PG, Murakami C, Jin Z, Warren D, Momtaz P, Hoppensteadt D, et al. Multi-institutional use of defibrotide in 88 patients after stem cell transplantation with severe venoocclusive disease and multisystem organ failure: response without significant toxicity in a high-risk population and factors predictive of outcome. Blood 2002;100:4337–43.

[36] Corbacioglu S, Greil J, Peters C, Wulffraat N, Laes HJ, Dilloo D, et al. Defibrotide in the treatment of children with veno-occlusive disease (VOD): a retrospective multicentre study demonstrates therapeutic efficacy upon early intervention. Bone Marrow Transplant 2004;33:189–95.

[37] Martinez MT, Bucher CH, Stussi G, Heim D, Buser A, Tsakiris DA, et al. Transplant-associated microangiopathy (TAM) in recipients of allogeneic hematopoietic stem cell transplants. Bone Marrow Transplant 2005;36:993-1000.

[38] Rosenthal RA, Chukwuogo NA, Ocasio VH, Kahng KU. Cyclosporine inhibits endothelial cell prostacyclin production. J Surg Res 1989;46:593–6.

[39] Voss BL, Hamilton KK, Samara EN, McKee PA. Cyclosporine suppression of endothelial prostacyclin generation: a possible mechanism for nephrotoxicity. Transplantation 1988;45:793–6.

[40] Lau DC, Wong KL, Hwang WS. Cyclosporine toxicity on cultured rat microvascular endothelial cells. Kidney Int 1989;35:604–13.

[41] Benigni A, Morigi M, Perico N, Zoja C, Amuchastegui CS, Piccinelli A, et al. The acute effect of FK506 and cyclosporine on endothelial cell function and renal vascular resistance. Transplantation 1992;54:775–80.

[42] Nitta K, Uchida K, Tsutsui T, Horita S, Hayashi T, Ozu H, et al. Cyclosporin A induces glomerular endothelial cell injury in vitro. Acta Pathol Jpn 1993;43:367–71.
[43] Azizian M, Ramenaden ER, Shah G, Wilasrusmee C, Bruch D, Kittur DS. Augmentation of ischemia/reperfusion injury to endothelial cells by cyclosporine A. Am Surg 2004;70:438–42.
[44] Nacar A, Kiyici H, Ogus E, Zagyapan R, Demirhan B, Ozdemir H, et al. Ultrastructural examination of glomerular and tubular changes in renal allografts with cyclosporine toxicity. Ren Fail 2006;28:543–7.
[45] Burke GW, Ciancio G, Cirocco R, Markou M, Olson L, Contreras N, et al. Microangiopathy in kidney and simultaneous pancreas/kidney recipients treated with tacrolimus: evidence of endothelin and cytokine involvement. Transplantation 1999;68:1336–42.
[46] Cutler C, Henry NL, Magee C, Li S, Kim HT, Alyea E, et al. Sirolimus and thrombotic microangiopathy after allogeneic hematopoietic stem cell transplantation. Biol Blood Marrow Transplant 2005;11:551–7.
[47] Couriel DR, Saliba R, Escalon MP, Hsu Y, Ghosh S, Ippoliti C, et al. Sirolimus in combination with tacrolimus and corticosteroids for the treatment of resistant chronic graftversus-host disease. Br J Haematol 2005;130:409–17.
[48] Fortin MC, Raymond MA, Madore F, Fugere JA, Paquet M, St-Louis G, et al. Increased risk of thrombotic microangiopathy in patients receiving a cyclosporine-sirolimus combination. Am J Transplant 2004;4:946–52.
[49] Erbey F, Bayram I, Yilmaz S, Tanyeli A. The overwiev of diagnostic criteria and treatment options of transplantation associated thrombotic microangiopathy with two case reports. Int J Hematol Oncol 2010;20(2):110-114.
[50] Erbey F, Bayram I, Kuskonmaz B, Yilmaz S, Cetin M, Uckan D, Tanyeli A. Thrombotic microangiopathy in allogeneic stem cell transplantation in childhood. Exp Clin Transplant 2010;8(3):237-244.
[51] Pettitt AR, Clark RE. Thrombotic microangiopathy following bone marrow transplantation. Bone Marrow Transplant 1994;14:495-504.
[52] Furlong T, Storb R, Anasetti C, Appelbaum FR, Deeg HJ, Doney K, et al. Clinical outcome after conversion to FK 506 (tacrolimus) therapy for acute graft-versus-host disease resistant to cyclosporine or for cyclosporine-associated toxicities. Bone Marrow Transplant 2000;26:985–91.
[53] Rock G, Shumak KH, Sutton DM, Busdkard NA, Nair RC. Cryosupernatant as replacement fluid for plasma exchange in thrombotic thrombocytopenic purpura. Members of the Canadian Apheresis Group. Br J Haematol 1996;94:383–6.
[54] Ho VT, Cutler C, Carter S, Martin P, Adams R, Horowitz M, et al. Blood and marrow transplant clinical trials network toxicity committee consensus summary: thrombotic microangiopathy after hematopoietic stem cell transplantation. Biol Blood Marrow Transplant 2005;11:571–5.
[55] Elliott MA, Nichols WL, Plumhoff EA, Ansell SM, Dispenzieri A, Gastineau DA, et al. Posttransplantation thrombotic thrombocytopenic purpura: a single-center experience and a contemporary review. Mayo Clin Proc 2003;78:421–30.
[56] Rizvi MA, Vesely SK, George JN, Chandler L, Duvall D, Smith JW, et al. Complications of plasma exchange in 71 consecutive patients treated for clinically suspected

thrombotic thrombocytopenic purpura-hemolytic-uremic syndrome. Transfusion 2000;40:896–901.
[57] McMinn JR, Thomas IA, Terrell DR, Duvall D, Vesely SK, George JN. Complications of plasma exchange in thrombotic thrombocytopenic purpura-hemolytic uremic syndrome: a study of 78 additional patients. Transfusion 2003;43:415–6.
[58] Howard MA, Williams LA, Terrell DR, Duvall D, Vesely SK, Georgre JN. Complications of plasma exchange in patients treated for clinically suspected thrombotic thrombocytopenic purpura-hemolytic uremic syndrome. Transfusion 2006;46:154–6.
[59] George JN, Selby GB. Thrombotic microangiopathy after allogeneic bone marrow transplantation: a pathologic abnormality associated with diverse clinical syndromes. Bone Marrow Transplant 2004;33:1073–4.
[60] Schroder H. Defibrotide protects endothelial cells, but not L929 tumour cells, from tumour necrosis factor-a-mediated cytotoxicity. J Pharm Pharmocol 1995;47:250–2.
[61] Corti P, Uderzo C, Tagliabue A, Della Volpe A, Annaloro C, Tagliaferri E, et al. Defibrotide as a promising treatment for thrombotic thrombocytopenic purpura in patients undergoing bone marrow transplantation. Bone Marrow Transplant 2002;29:542–3.
[62] Wolff D, Wilhelm S, Hahn J, Gentilini C, Hilgendorf I, Steiner B, et al. Replacement of calcineurin inhibitors with daclizumab in patients with transplantation-associated microangiopathy or renal insufficiency associated with graft-versushost disease. Bone Marrow Transplant 2006;38:445–51.
[63] Au WY, Ma ES, Lee TL, Ha SY, Fung AT, Lie AK, et al. Successful treatment of thrombotic microangiopathy after haematopoietic stem cell transplantation with rituximab. Br J Haematol 2007;137:475–8.
[64] Takatsuka H, Takemoto Y, Iwata N, Suehiro A, Hamano T, Okamoto T, et al. Oral eicosapentaenoic acid for complications of bone marrow transplantation. Bone Marrow Transplant 2001;28:769–74.
[65] Kajiume T, Nagita A, Yoshimi S, Kobayashi K, Kataoka N. A case of hemolytic-uremic syndrome improved with nitric oxide. Bone Marrow Transplant 2000;25:109–10.
[66] Kobbe G, Schneider P, Rohr U, Fenk R, Neumann F, Aivado M, et al. Treatment of severe steroid refractory acute graft-versus-host disease with infliximab, a chimeric human/mouse anti-TNFalpha antibody. Bone Marrow Transplant 2001;28:47–9.
[67] Couriel D, Saliba R, Hicks K, Ippoliti C, de Lima M, Hosing C, et al. Tumor necrosis factor-a blockade for the treatment of acute GVHD. Blood 2004;104:649–54.
[68] Patriarca F, Sperotto A, Damiani D, Morreale G, Bonifazi F, Olivieri A, et al. Infliximab treatment for steroid refractory acute graft versus host disease. Haematologica 2004;89:1352–9.
[69] Uberti JP, Ayash L, Ratanatharathorn V, Silver S, Reynolds C, Becker M, et al. Pilot trial on the use of etanercept and methylprednisolone as primary treatment for acute graftversus-host disease. Biol Blood Marrow Transplant 2005;11:680–7.
[70] Kennedy GA, Butler J, Western R. Combination antithymocyte globulin and soluble TNFalpha inhibitor (etanercept) +/_ mycophenolate mofetil for treatment of steroid refractory acute graft-versus-host disease. Bone Marrow Transplant 2006;37:1143–7.

[71] Busca A, Locatelli F, Marmont F, Ceretto C, Falda M. Recombinant human soluble tumor necrosis factor receptor fusion protein as treatment for steroid refractory graft-versushost disease following allogeneic hematopoietic stem cell transplantation. Am J Hematol 2007;82:45–52.

[72] Ambrosi P, Aillaud MF, Habib G, Kreitmann B, Metras D, Luccioni R, et al. Fluvastatin decreases soluble thrombomodulin in cardiac transplant recipients. Thromb Haemost 2000;84:46–8.

[73] Chello M, Carassiti M, Agro F, Mastroroberto P, Pugliese G, Colonna D, et al. Simvastatin blunts the increase of circulating adhesion molecules after coronary artery bypass surgery with cardiopulmonary bypass. J Cardiothorac Vasc Anesth 2004;18:605–9.

[74] Chello M, Goffredo C, Patti G, Candura D, Melfi R, Mastrobuoni S, et al. Effects of atorvastatin on arterial endothelial function in coronary bypass surgery. Eur J Cardiothorac Surg 2005;28:805–10.

[75] Patti G, Chello M, Pasceri V, Colonna D, Nusca A, Miglionico M, et al. Protection from procedural myocardial injury by atorvastatin is associated with lower levels of adhesion molecules after percutaneous coronary intervention: results from the ARMYDA-CAMs (Atorvastatin for Reduction of Myocardial Damage during Angioplasty-Cell Adhesion Molecules) substudy. J Am Coll Cardiol 2006;48:1560–6.

[76] Boehme MW, Gao IK, Norden C, Lemmel EM. Decrease in circulating endothelial cell adhesion molecule and thrombomodulin levels during oral iloprost treatment in rheumatoid arthritis patients: preliminary results. Rheumatol Int 2006;26:340–7.

[77] Wilasrusmee C, Ondocin P, Bruch D, Shah G, Kittur S, Wilarusmee S, et al. Amelioration of cyclosporine A effect on microvasculature by endothelin inhibitor. Surgery 2003;134:384–9.

[78] Bohm F, Settergren M, Gonon AT, Pernow J. The endothelin-1 receptor antagonist bosentan protects against ischaemia/reperfusion-induced endothelial dysfunction in humans. Clin Sci (Lond) 2005;108:357–63.

[79] Yamshita T, Shoge M, Oda E, Yamamoto Y, Giddings JC, Kashiwagi S, et al. The free-radical scavenger, edaravone, augments NO release from vascular cells and platelets after laser-induced, acute endothelial injury in vivo. Platelets 2006;17:201–6.

[80] Sueishi K, Mishima K, Makino K, Itoh Y, Tsuruya K, Hirakata H, et al. Protection by a radical scavenger edaravone against cisplatin-induced nephrotoxicity in rats. Eur J Pharmacol 2002;451:203–8.

[81] Ruutu T, Hermans I, Niederwieser D, Gratwohl A, Kiehl M, Volin L, et al. Thrombotic thrombocytopenic purpura after allogeneic stem cell transplantation: a survey of the European Group for Blood and Marrow Transplantation (EBMT). Br J Haematol 2002;118:1112–9.

[82] Uderzo C, Bonanomi S, Busca A, Renoldi M, Ferrari P, Iacobelli M, et al. Risk factors and severe outcome in thrombotic microangiopathy after allogeneic hematopoietic stem cell transplantation. Transplantation 2006;82:638–44.

Part 2

Eclampsia-Associated Microangiopathy

3

Renal Effects of Preeclampsia

Kuang-Yu Jen and Zoltan G. Laszik
University of California, San Francisco, USA

1. Introduction

Dramatic hemodynamic alterations occur during a normal, healthy pregnancy with the kidneys playing a major role to ensure that these adaptive changes occur properly. Therefore, it is not surprising that a significant number of women may develop new onset renal dysfunction or exacerbation of preexisting renal disease during pregnancy. Perhaps the most commonly encountered gestational disorder is hypertension, which can lead to significant complications for both the mother and the fetus when left untreated. A variety of factors may cause or contribute to the development or worsening of hypertension during pregnancy; nevertheless, clinically, hypertensive disorders of pregnancy can be divided into four major categories as recommended by the National High Blood Pressure Education Program Working Group on High Blood Pressure in Pregnancy: preeclampsia, chronic/preexisting hypertension, preeclampsia superimposed upon chronic hypertension, and gestational hypertension [1]. Of particular importance in defining these categories is the time of onset of hypertension during pregnancy, whether the women had preexisting hypertension prior to pregnancy, and whether proteinuria is present. Hypertension prior to pregnancy or occurring before 20 weeks of gestation indicates chronic/preexisting hypertension while hypertension occurring after 20 weeks of gestation but without proteinuria defines gestational hypertension. Preeclamspia is gestational hypertension with the additional feature of proteinuria. Of these hypertensive disorders of pregnancy, preeclampsia is the most common and can cause devastating systemic consequences including substantial renal injury. In this chapter, we discuss the pathologic manifestations and molecular pathologenesis of preeclampsia with a special emphasis on the renal effects of this disease.

2. Clinical definition, epidemiology, and presentation

Preeclamspia is a systemic syndrome of pregnancy defined by new onset hypertension (systolic ≥140 mmHg or diastolic ≥90 mmHg) and proteinuria of ≥0.3 grams per 24-hour occurring after 20 weeks of gestation in a previously normotensive woman [1, 2]. The incidence of preeclampsia is somewhat variable depending on the study population, but estimates generally range from 3 to 7% of all pregnancies [3-6], making it the leading cause of maternal and fetal morbidity and mortality and perhaps the most frequently encountered glomerular disease worldwide. Many factors have been associated with an increased risk of developing preeclampsia including prior history or family history of preeclampsia, nulliparity, multigestational pregnancy, long time interval between pregnancies, obesity, age >40 years, diabetes mellitus, and preexisting history of other medical conditions such as chronic hypertension and renal disease, among others [7-10].

Preeclampsia can be subdivided into mild and severe, with severe forms exhibiting more prominent signs and symptoms of end-organ damage that may result in life-threatening disease. Multiple organ systems may be affected in severe preeclampsia including dysfunction of the central nervous system (i.e. blurred vision, altered mental status, severe headache, cerebrovascular accident), liver (i.e. elevated serum transaminases), cardiovascular system (i.e. systolic blood pressure ≥160 mm Hg or diastolic ≥110 mm Hg), lungs (i.e. pulmonary edema, cyanosis), and/or kidneys (i.e. proteinuria of ≥5 grams in 24 hours, oliguria of <500 mL in 24 hours) [1, 11]. Other notable disease features include potential manifestation of microangiopathic hemolytic anemia, thrombocytopenia, and severe fetal growth restriction [12]. Preeclampsia with concurrent symptom of grand mal seizures with no other attributable cause supports the diagnosis of eclampsia. HELLP syndrome, a life-threatening variant of preeclampsia, may develop in approximately 10 to 20% of women with severe preeclampsia [13]. The additional laboratory findings of microangiopathic hemolysis, elevated liver enzymes, and a low platelet count (thrombocytopenia) establish the diagnosis of HELLP syndrome and represent more prominent and systemic end-organ injury.

Typically, women with preeclampsia display mild proteinuria; however, nephrotic range proteinuria and slight hematuria may be seen in severe preeclampsia and represents a significantly increased risk for complications [11]. Although edema can be present in preeclamptic patients, normal pregnancies often will induce edema, making this finding unreliable for the diagnosis of preeclampsia. A dramatic decrease in glomerular filtration rate may occur in preeclampsia although serum creatinine is generally close to baseline levels or may be slightly elevated. Acute renal failure is highly unusual. Other potential clinical features include hyperuricemia and hypercalciuria.

Since renal diseases, especially those of glomerular origin, often present with hypertension and proteinuria, the clinical differential diagnosis of preeclampsia is broad and includes various glomerular diseases. Chronic glomerulonephritis, minimal change nephrotic syndrome, focal segmental glomerulosclerosis, membranous nephropathy, postinfectious glomerulonephritis, diabetic nephropathy, and sickle cell nephropathy should be considered. In severe cases of preeclampsia with significant microangiopathic hemolytic anemia and thrombocytopenia, hemolytic-uremic syndrome (HUS) and thrombotic thrombocytopenic purpura (TTP) should also be included in the differential diagnosis [12].

3. Pathologic findings

Although preeclampsia is a clinical diagnosis based on new onset hypertension and proteinuria, as mentioned earlier, the specificity of these features is low and a renal biopsy may be helpful to confirm the suspicion of preeclampsia. Since many other forms of renal diseases may arise during pregnancy, the utility of the renal biopsy is also to exclude (or include) other pathologic processes of the kidney that may mimic preeclampsia clinically.

Typically, preeclampsia manifests morphologically as thrombotic microangiopathy (TMA) on renal biopsy, a pattern of renal injury commonly seen in association with endothelial cell injury. It should be stressed that TMA is a histologic and ultrastructural pattern that develops in response to renal injury and is not a specific disease. Many etiologies of TMA exist, including but not limited to TTP, HUS, malignant hypertension, scleroderma/systemic sclerosis, drugs/medications, antibody-mediated rejection (in allografts), and preeclampsia/eclampsia. Although a few subtle morphologic features appear to be seen more often in renal biopsies from patients with preeclampsia (discussed below); overall, these findings remain relatively non-specific and are not entirely reliable as morphologic indicators to distinguish preeclampsia from other etiologies of TMA.

3.1 Light microscopy

Since TMA is a disease that results from small vessel endothelial cell injury, the major morphologic findings reside within the glomeruli and/or the arterioles, the hallmark of which is that of fibrin platelet thrombi within these small vessels. However, unlike other etiologies of TMA, preeclampsia typically does not exhibit platelet fibrin thrombi within glomerular capillary lumina. Instead, the most characteristic glomerular feature of preeclampsia is that of prominent glomerular endothelial cell swelling, termed endotheliosis. This process results in occlusion of the glomerular capillary lumina without an appreciable increase in cellularity and generally gives the glomerular tuft a lobularly accentuated appearance (Figure 1). Overall, glomerular volume is slightly increased, yet since glomerular cellularity remains relatively unchanged, an impression of somewhat hypocellular glomeruli that take on a "bloodless" appearance is classically described in preeclampsia due to the endotheliosis. Variable degrees of mesangiolysis are commonly noted, but significant mesangial matrix widening or mesangial hypercellularity is not typically present. The glomerular tuft may also often exhibit capillary loop wrinkling with mild collapse/shrinkage of the glomerular tuft characteristic of acute ischemic changes. This feature is frequently seen in association with severe arteriolar changes in the afferent arteriole and most likely is due to hypoperfusion of the glomeruli from compromised arteriolar blood flow. Prominence of the visceral epithelial cells may be observed due to proteinuria; however, this finding may be quite variable and may, to a certain degree, depend on the severity of the proteinuria. The glomeruli can be either segmentally or globally involved, and the kidney may be focally or diffusely affected, depending on the severity of the disease.

In chronic stages of TMA (including preeclampsia), the glomeruli typically display extensive glomerular capillary basement membrane replication, a feature similar to the "tram tracking" seen in membranoproliferative glomerulonephritis (MPGN) or in transplant nephropathy of renal allografts. Therefore, this morphologic feature is non-specific and is a consequence of long term glomerular endothelial cell injury. However, unlike MPGN where subendothelial immune deposits are present on immunofluorescence and electron microscopy and sometimes can even be appreciated on light microscopy, chronic stages of TMA show no evidence of an immune complex-mediated process. In allografts, chronic changes of TMA are indistinguishable from transplant glomerulopathy.

Arteriolar pathology is also often present along with the glomerular changes. Arterioles commonly display striking intimal swelling/edema with substantial luminal closure. Fibrin platelet thrombi and/or schisctocytes may be seen within the narrowed lumina. As mentioned earlier, this feature may markedly compromise afferent blood flow into the glomeruli resulting in glomerular ischemia. In the subacute phase, the intimal swelling becomes replaced by scarring. At first, appreciable numbers of cells are seen within the early intimal concentric scar giving an "onion skin" appearance. As scarring becomes more established, intimal fibroplasia sets in and is essentially indistinguishable from severe arteriolosclerosis seen in other etiologies of chronic vascular disease.

3.2 Immunofluorescence microscopy

Immunofluorescence microscopy shows no specific features for TMA or TMA as a result of preeclampsia. Fibrin, IgM, and to a lesser extent, complement components, may be positive within glomeruli along the capillary walls, in the mesangium, and in arterioles especially during acute stages of the disease, the latter of which corresponds to intravascular fibrin platelet thrombi seen on light microscopic evaluation [14-16]. The immunofluorescence intensity somewhat correlates to the severity/activity of the disease [15]. Although TMA can show fibrin positivity within the glomerular intracapillary lumina, preeclampsia rarely displays this finding. IgG is minimally positive if present, and IgA is usually negative.

3.3 Electron microscopy

Similar to the light and immunofluorescence microscopic findings, ultrastructural characteristics of TMA are similar regardless of the etiology. In the acute phase, electron microscopic examination of renal tissue from patients with TMA (including those with preeclampsia) reveal thickening of the glomerular capillary walls due to a combination of subendothelial widening, endothelial cell swelling, and occasional mesangial cell interposition. Often, the widened subendothelial space, represented as an expanded lamina rara interna, takes on a pale and flocculent appearance with irregular collections of slightly electron-dense material, typically without appreciable fibrin. Similar material can occasionally be seen within the mesangium, resulting in mesangial prominence with slight mesangial cell swelling. Electron-dense immuno-type deposits should be absent, and if present, should prompt further investigation into an immune complex-mediated process instead of or concurrent with TMA. As mentioned above, one slightly more distinguishing feature of preeclampsia is that of endotheliosis or endothelial cell swelling, which can be observed occluding much of the glomerular capillary lumina in severe cases (Figure 2). The endothelial cells in this instance lose their characteristic fenestrations. Although rarely seen in preeclampsia, intracapillary thrombi containing amorphous osmiophilic material admixed with fibrin, platelets, deformed red blood cells, and inflammatory cells can be present in other forms of TMA. Finally, podocyte foot processes often show at least focal, if not widespread, effacement.

In chronic stages, nonspecific glomerular capillary basement membrane wrinkling and thickening may be appreciated. Often, new glomerular basement membrane material is also present giving rise to basement membrane reduplication and architectural "complexity", features similar to that seen in transplant glomerulopathy in allograft kidney biopsies. Variable mesangial cell interposition can be observed.

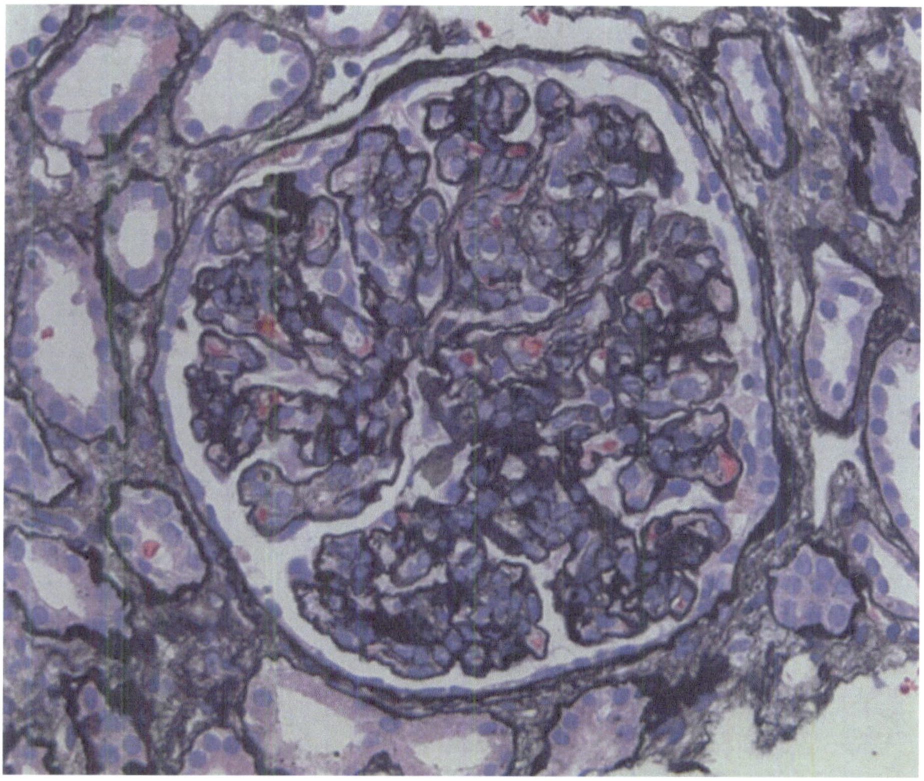

Fig. 1. Preeclampsia, light microscopy. The glomerular capillary tufts are distended with closure of the capillary lumina due to swollen endothelial cells. The glomerular appearance is slightly lobular. (Jones' methenamine silver, x400) (Courtesy of Dr. Patrick Walker and Nephropath, Little Rock, AK).

4. Pathogenesis

Microvascular endothelial cell injury appears to play a central role in the pathogenesis of preeclampsia. Therefore, as expected, end organ damage is generally directed towards organ systems highly dependent on the microvasculature for normal function including the kidney, liver, and central nervous system (including the eyes), among others. In order to fully comprehend the pathogenesis and renal consequences of preeclampsia, an understanding of renal physiology is required.

4.1 Renal physiology

The kidneys act as filters that eliminate waste products within the blood, and thus, receive up to 25% of the cardiac output. To accomplish this function, systemic blood flow enters the kidneys and is directed into the glomeruli through the afferent arterioles. Filtration occurs through the glomerular capillary loops, which constitute the glomerular filtration barrier (GFB) and consist of the glomerular capillary basement membrane (GBM) flanked by visceral epithelial cells (also known as podocytes) on the side of the Bowman space and glomerular capillary endothelial cells along the glomerular capillary lumina (Figure 3). The glomerular ultrafiltrate travels from the glomerular capillary lumina, through the endothelial cell fenestrations, through the GBM, and finally through the slit diaphragms between the podocyte foot processes, into the Bowman space. The integrity of the GFB prevents leakage of serum proteins into the Bowman space. However, when any component of the GFB is compromised, proteinuria arises.

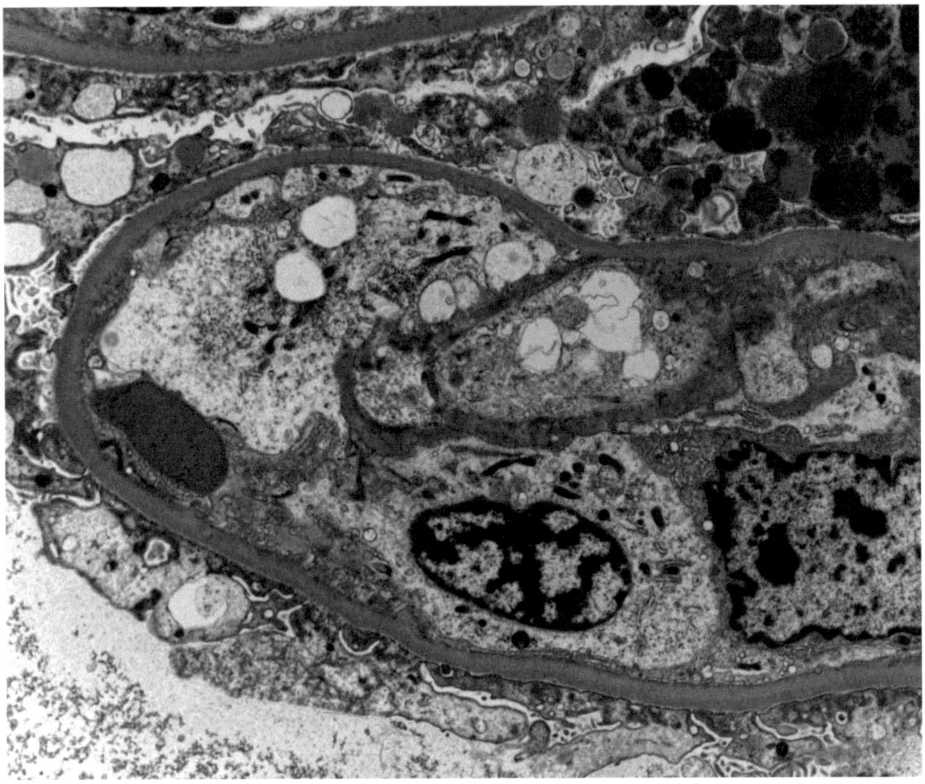

Fig. 2. Characteristic ultrastructural findings of preeclampsia. The glomerular capillary endothelial cells are swollen with occlusion of the capillary lumina. Note the significant effacement of the foot processes and the numerous protein resorption droplets within the visceral epithelial cells. (Electron microscopy, original magnification x4,800)

The glomerular consequences of preeclampsia can be understood in terms of disruption of the GFB through glomerular capillary endothelial cell injury. Not only does endothelial damage result in endotheliosis and loss of endothelial cell fenestrations, the podocytes are disrupted as well since these remarkably specialized cells are highly dependent on signals derived from the glomerular endothelial cells to maintain foot process structure and the slit diaphragms. Ultimately, glomerular endothelial cell injury causes the breakdown of multiple components of the GFB, which leads to proteinuria and hypertension. Arteriolar endothelial injury also occurs in preeclampsia and may induce significant narrowing of arteriolar lumina. Consequently, glomerular filtration is compromised and results in glomerular hypoperfusion and diminished glomerular filtration rate with renal compensation manifesting as elevated blood pressure.

4.2 Molecular mechanism of preeclampsia

Recently, extraordinary progress has been made in adding to our understanding of the molecular mechanism of preeclampsia. As mentioned earlier, the root of preeclampsia as a disease process lies in microvascular endothelial cell injury. Much of the data point to abnormal placentation or other causes of aberrant placental vascular development as the initiating event, which leads to placental hypoxia and subsequently triggers the release of placenta-derived factors into the maternal circulation. Consequently, these factors, most of which have antiangiogenic properties, cause damage to the microvascular endothelium by altering local angiogenic and vasodilatory signals.

Several circulating factors have been implicated in the pathogenesis of preeclampsia, perhaps the best studied of which is soluble Flt-1 (sFlt1). This secreted form of vascular endothelial growth factor (VEGF) receptor-1 is able to bind and sequester angiogenic factors such as VEGFA and placental growth factor (PIGF), acting as an endogenous inhibitor of VEGF-receptor signaling. In preeclampsia, excessive levels of sFlt1, thought to originate from the placenta, appears to disrupt VEGF-receptor signaling, which is essential for the maintenance of endothelial health (Figure 3). As a result, tipping the endothelial environment towards an antiangiogenic state leads to generalized damage to the endothelium. In the glomeruli, glomerular endothelial cell injury results in disruption of the GFB with clinical consequences to the kidney as described earlier. In support of this mechanism of preeclampsia, several studies have shown that women with established preeclampsia display elevated levels of serum sFlt1 and that this increase may occur even before the onset of hypertension [17, 18]. Additionally, animal models overexpressing sFlt1 produce clinical signs and glomerular lesions reminiscent of human preeclampsia [17] . Similar observations have been reported in rodents when neutralizing antibodies to VEGFA are administered [19]. On the other hand, exogenous administration of VEGFA alleviates this preeclampsia-like phenotype in rats without apparent harm to the fetus [20]. Likewise, renal damage induced in mice by adenoviral overexpression of sFlt1 is alleviated by reducing circulating sFlt1 through co-expression of VEGF [21].

Some studies indicate that soluble endoglin (sEng) may act in a similar manner as sFlt1 in the pathogenesis of preeclampsia. Just as in the case of sFlt1, sEng likely produced by the placenta is also elevated in the sera of women with preeclampsia and correlates with disease severity [22, 23]. Interestingly, although overexpression of sEng alone in animal models gives only mild proteinuria when compared to sFlt1 overexpression, concurrent elevation of these factors leads to severe preeclampsia with evidence of HELLP syndrome [22]. The effects of sEng may be propagated through the disruption of transforming growth factor beta 1 (TGFB1) signaling with subsequent impairment of TGFB1-mediated activation of endothelial nitric oxide synthetase (eNOS) (Figure 3) [22]. Since eNOS is of prime importance in regulating vascular tone and also displays angiogenic properties, abrogation of eNOS as a result of elevated sEng levels induces endothelial cell injury and defects in vasodilatation. Of note, hypoxia up-regulates the placental expression of endoglin [24]. Therefore, placental hypoxia due to abnormal placentation may give rise to sEng elevation, and in combination with other antiangiogenic factors like sFlt1, may result in the development of preeclampsia or HELLP syndrome.

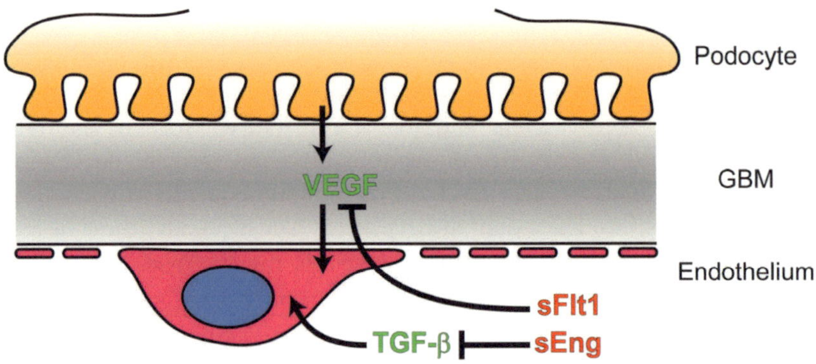

Fig. 3. VEGF produced by the podocytes is required to maintain healthy endothelial cells. Circulating sFlt1, likely originating from the placenta, is able to bind and sequester VEGF, resulting in endothelial cell damage. Similarly, the pro-endothelial effects of circulating TGF-β are inhibited by sEng, leading to endothelial injury.

5. Prognosis and treatment

At this time, delivery of the neonate and placenta is the only definitive cure of preeclampsia; however, fetal morbidity and mortality is highly dependent on the gestational age at the time of delivery. Therefore, a crucial decision must be made to weigh the benefits of delivery for the mother against the risks of prematurity for the neonate. Generally, quick resolution of both hypertension and proteinuria follows delivery.

If delivery is not a viable option, management with antihypertensive medications and prophylactic seizure treatment with intravenous magnesium sulfate may be initiated [25-27]. If preterm delivery prior to 34 weeks is considered, betamethasone is commonly given to the mother to hasten fetal lung development [28]. In severe cases of preeclampsia/eclampsia where preterm delivery is not a viable option, maternal symptoms of significant microangiopathic hemolytic anemia, thrombocytopenia, renal failure, and/or neurologic abnormalities may be treated with plasma exchange with variable benefit [12].

Currently, treatment for preeclampsia is largely supportive, requiring careful obstetric management. As we make significant progress in elucidating the molecular mechanisms of preeclampsia, the hope of future targeted therapies to ameliorate or even prevent the development of preeclampsia appears to inch closer to reality. Given the immense health impact of preeclampsia due to its high worldwide prevalence, progress in this field has the potential to greatly improve global women's health in a relatively short period of time.

6. References

[1] *Report of the National High Blood Pressure Education Program Working Group on High Blood Pressure in Pregnancy.* Am J Obstet Gynecol, 2000. 183(1): p. S1-S22.

[2] Roberts, J.M., et al., *Summary of the NHLBI Working Group on Research on Hypertension During Pregnancy.* Hypertension, 2003. 41(3): p. 437-45.

[3] Stillman, I.E. and S.A. Karumanchi, *The glomerular injury of preeclampsia.* J Am Soc Nephrol, 2007. 18(8): p. 2281-4.

[4] Saftlas, A.F., et al., *Epidemiology of preeclampsia and eclampsia in the United States, 1979-1986.* Am J Obstet Gynecol, 1990. 163(2): p. 460-5.
[5] Sibai, B.M., et al., *Risk factors for preeclampsia in healthy nulliparous women: a prospective multicenter study. The National Institute of Child Health and Human Development Network of Maternal-Fetal Medicine Units.* Am J Obstet Gynecol, 1995. 172(2 Pt 1): p. 642-8.
[6] Zhang, J., S. Meikle, and A. Trumble, *Severe maternal morbidity associated with hypertensive disorders in pregnancy in the United States.* Hypertens Pregnancy, 2003. 22(2): p. 203-12.
[7] Duckitt, K. and D. Harrington, *Risk factors for pre-eclampsia at antenatal booking: systematic review of controlled studies.* BMJ, 2005. 330(7491): p. 565.
[8] Xiong, X., W.D. Fraser, and N.N. Demianczuk, *History of abortion, preterm, term birth, and risk of preeclampsia: a population-based study.* Am J Obstet Gynecol, 2002. 187(4): p. 1013-8.
[9] Nilsson, E., et al., *The importance of genetic and environmental effects for pre-eclampsia and gestational hypertension: a family study.* BJOG, 2004. 111(3): p. 200-6.
[10] van Rijn, B.B., et al., *Outcomes of subsequent pregnancy after first pregnancy with early-onset preeclampsia.* Am J Obstet Gynecol, 2006. 195(3): p. 723-8.
[11] Lindheimer, M.D., S.J. Taler, and F.G. Cunningham, *Hypertension in pregnancy.* J Am Soc Hypertens, 2010. 4(2): p. 68-78.
[12] McMinn, J.R. and J.N. George, *Evaluation of women with clinically suspected thrombotic thrombocytopenic purpura-hemolytic uremic syndrome during pregnancy.* J Clin Apher, 2001. 16(4): p. 202-9.
[13] Karumanchi, S.A., et al., *Preeclampsia: a renal perspective.* Kidney Int, 2005. 67(6): p. 2101-13.
[14] Gonzalo, A., et al., *Hemolytic uremic syndrome with hypocomplementemia and deposits of IgM and C3 in the involved renal tissue.* Clin Nephrol, 1981. 16(4): p. 193-9.
[15] Petrucco, O.M., et al., *Immunofluorescent studies in renal biopsies in pre-eclampsia.* Br Med J, 1974. 1(5906): p. 473-6.
[16] Gaber, L.W., B.H. Spargo, and M.D. Lindheimer, *Renal pathology in pre-eclampsia.* Baillieres Clin Obstet Gynaecol, 1994. 8(2): p. 443-68.
[17] Maynard, S.E., et al., *Excess placental soluble fms-like tyrosine kinase 1 (sFlt1) may contribute to endothelial dysfunction, hypertension, and proteinuria in preeclampsia.* J Clin Invest, 2003. 111(5): p. 649-58.
[18] Levine, R.J., et al., *Circulating angiogenic factors and the risk of preeclampsia.* N Engl J Med, 2004. 350(7): p. 672-83.
[19] Sugimoto, H., et al., *Neutralization of circulating vascular endothelial growth factor (VEGF) by anti-VEGF antibodies and soluble VEGF receptor 1 (sFlt-1) induces proteinuria.* J Biol Chem, 2003. 278(15): p. 12605-8.
[20] Li, Z., et al., *Recombinant vascular endothelial growth factor 121 attenuates hypertension and improves kidney damage in a rat model of preeclampsia.* Hypertension, 2007. 50(4): p. 686-92.
[21] Bergmann, A., et al., *Reduction of circulating soluble Flt-1 alleviates preeclampsia-like symptoms in a mouse model.* J Cell Mol Med, 2010. 14(6B): p. 1857-67.
[22] Venkatesha, S., et al., *Soluble endoglin contributes to the pathogenesis of preeclampsia.* Nat Med, 2006. 12(6): p. 642-9.

[23] Levine, R.J., et al., *Soluble endoglin and other circulating antiangiogenic factors in preeclampsia.* N Engl J Med, 2006. 355(10): p. 992-1005.
[24] Yinon, Y., et al., *Severe intrauterine growth restriction pregnancies have increased placental endoglin levels: hypoxic regulation via transforming growth factor-beta 3.* Am J Pathol, 2008. 172(1): p. 77-85.
[25] Sibai, B.M., *Magnesium sulfate prophylaxis in preeclampsia: Lessons learned from recent trials.* Am J Obstet Gynecol, 2004. 190(6): p. 1520-6.
[26] Lain, K.Y. and J.M. Roberts, *Contemporary concepts of the pathogenesis and management of preeclampsia.* JAMA, 2002. 287(24): p. 3183-6.
[27] Wagner, L.K., *Diagnosis and management of preeclampsia.* Am Fam Physician, 2004. 70(12): p. 2317-24.
[28] Szabo, I., M. Vizer, and T. Ertl, *Fetal betamethasone treatment and neonatal outcome in preeclampsia and intrauterine growth restriction.* Am J Obstet Gynecol, 2003. 189(6): p. 1812-3; author reply 1813.

Part 3

Diabetic Microangiopathy

4

Diabetic Microangiopathy – Etiopathogenesis, New Possibilities in Diagnostics and Management

Jarmila Vojtková, Miriam Čiljaková and Peter Bánovčin
Jessenius Faculty of Medicine in Martin, Department of Children and Adolescents
Slovakia

1. Introduction

Diabetic microangiopathy is characterized as a disorder of small vessels. It is one of the major chronic diabetic complications involving diabetic neuropathy, retinopathy and nephropathy (Adeghate et al., 2006). Its prevalence has rising tendency even in children population and is possitivelly associated with duration of diabetes mellitus.

Diabetic neuropathy affects peripheral nerves (sensory, motor, autonomic) so all organ systems can be affected. In childhood, subclinical forms are typical when no clinical symptoms are evident, however sensitive diagnostic methods can detect them. Later, autonomic and sensory-motor neuropathy is very common (see the classification in table 1). Some forms of diabetic neuropathy are presented in 40 - 90% of patients with diabetes duration ten years and more and even in 5% of patients after one year of diabetes diagnostics.

<table>
<tr><td colspan="4">Subclinical neuropathy</td></tr>
<tr><td rowspan="10">Clinical neuropathy</td><td rowspan="4">Symetric</td><td>Distal symetric neuropathy</td><td>sensoric
motoric
mixed</td></tr>
<tr><td colspan="2">Autonomic neuropathy</td></tr>
<tr><td colspan="2">Proximal symetric neuropathy</td></tr>
<tr><td colspan="2">Acute painful neuropathy</td></tr>
<tr><td rowspan="4">Asymetric</td><td colspan="2">Cranial neuropathy</td></tr>
<tr><td colspan="2">Peripheral mononeuropathy</td></tr>
<tr><td colspan="2">Radiculopathy</td></tr>
<tr><td colspan="2">Asymetric proximal motoric neuropathy</td></tr>
<tr><td colspan="3">Mixed</td></tr>
</table>

Table 1. Classification of diabetic neuropathy (Rybka, 2007)

Diabetic retinopathy is the most frequent cause of new cases of blindness among adults aged 20 - 74. It progresses from mild nonproliferative abnormalities characterized by increased vascular permeability to moderate and severe nonproliferative retinopathy characterized by vascular closure to proliferative retinopathy with typical new blood vessels growth (table 2). The prevalence of retinopathy is noticed in 2 - 7% of diabetic patients after two years, in 50% of patients after ten years and in 75% of patients after twenty and more years of diabetes duration.

Diabetic nephropathy is characterized by glomerular, tubular and mesangial damage accompanied by basement membrane thickening, mesangial expansion and hyalinisation of glomerular intercapillary connective tissue. In clinical practice, progressive kidney disease with proteinuria, hypertension and gradual decrease in renal functions is typical (table 3). Manifest nephropathy is presented in 30 - 35% of patients with diabetes duration over fifteen years.

	Eye background
Non-proliferative DR	
Mild	Microaneurysmas, microhemorrhages, intraretinal hemorrhage, venous abnormalities
Moderate	Vessel changes at macula area, hard exudates, „cotton" exudates
Severe	Intraretinal microvascular abnormalities (IRMA), retinal ischemia
Proliferative DR	
Beginning	Retinal or papilar neovascularisation
High risk	Traction amotio of retina, intravital hemorrhage
Diabetic maculopathy	Macular edema

Table 2. Clinical stages of diabetic retinopathy (DR) (Rybka, 2007)

	characteristics	**Urinary findings**
1. Latent stage (hyperfiltration-hypertrophic)	increase GF about 10 - 40%, ultrasound hypertrophic of kidneys, slightly enlargement of basal membrane	transitory microalbuminuria 30 - 100 mg/day, resp. 20 - 70 μg/min
2. Incipient diabetic nephropathy	decrease GF, common hypertension (mainly diastolic), progression in enlargement of basal membrane	permanent microalbuminuria 30 - 300 mg/day, resp. 20 - 200 μg/min
3. Manifest diabetic nephropathy	Next decrease GF, hypertension progression, sclerotisation of many glomerules	proteinuria >0,5 g/day
4. Chronic renal insufficiency even kidney failure	Terminal phase, uremia, dialysis necessary	proteinuria >0,5 g/day, serum creatinine > 200 μmol/l

Table 3. Clinical stages of diabetic nephropathy (Rybka, 2007)

2. Etiopathogenesis

The etiopathogenesis of diabetic microangiopathy is complex (Figure 1) and since now not completely understood. Long lasting hyperglycemia triggers the variety of pathways - non-enzymatic glycation of proteins, oxidative stress, polyole pathway and sorbitol production, activation of proteinkinase C production, decrease of vasodilatation products (nitric oxide, prostaglandines), decrease of myoinositol origin, change in $Na^{+}K^{+}$ATP-ase activity causing the endothelial damage and so the microangiopathy with disorder in many organ systems (Brownlee, 2005). However, according to the clinical experience, some patients with short duration and adequate compensation of diabetes mellitus (DM) have symptoms of microangiopathic complications, and some despite long duration and insufficient compensation do not suffer from any complications. That is why other factors have been considered as important in pathogenesis - genetic, epigenetic or immunologic factors (Villeneuve & Natarajan, 2010). According to Diabetes Control and Complication Trial (DCCT Research Group, 1993), important risk factors for microvascular complications are cigarette smoking and genetic susceptibility to hypertension at early stages of diabetes and poorer glycemic control, higher blood pressure and unfourable lipid profile at later stages.

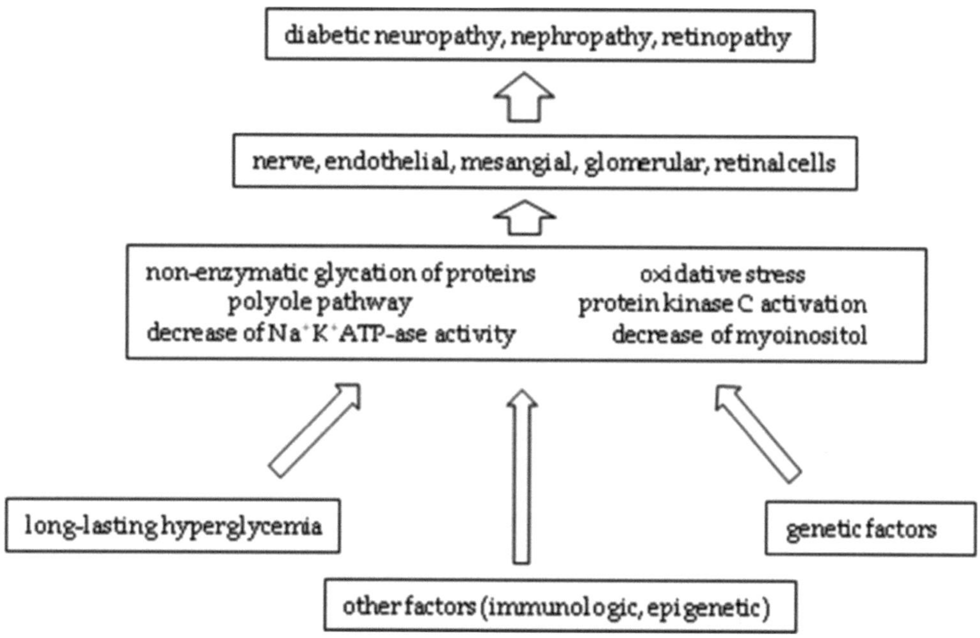

Fig. 1. Etiopathogenesis of diabetic microvascular complications

2.1 Advanced glycation end products

Advanced glycation end products (AGEP´s) are heterogeneous group of modified proteins, lipids and nucleic acids arisen within intracellular hyperglycemia by non-enzymatic Maillard reaction. The initial product of this reaction is called a Schiff base, which spontaneously rearranges itself into an Amadori product. These initial reactions are reversible depending on the concentration of glucose and reactants. Series of subsequent reactions (dehydratation, oxidation, reduction, other arrangements) lead to the formation of

AGEP´s. As precursors AGEP´s have typical ability for covalent crosslink formation between proteins, modified products have altered their structure and biological function (Peppa et al., 2003). Except endogenously formed AGEP´s, another source is exogenous like tobacco smoke and certain food. Nearly 10% of AGEP´s is absorbed through intestinal mucose from food like meat with high content of fat, meals prepared at high temperature (grilled, fried) (Klenoviscová et al., 2008). Contrary, fruit, vegetable and boiled, braised or steamed meals have noticably lower content of AGEP´s.

AGEP´s increase vascular permeability and production of growth factors and cytokines. They can modify extracellular matrix by changing its structure, solubility and charge leading to cummulation of collagen, fibronectin or laminin. Abnormalities in glomerular extracellular matrix lead to higher proliferation of mesangial cells and to increase in glomerular permeability which correlates with microalbuminuria (Cvetkovic et al., 2009). Glycated collagen can change the filtration abilities of glomerular basement membrane and can increase the binding of circulating plasmatic proteins.

Receptors for AGEP´s (RAGE) were found on vascular endothelial cells, macrophages, mesangial cells or smooth muscle cells. Interaction between AGEP´s and RAGE causes increase of oxidative stress, activation of transcriptional factor NFκB and expression of inflammatory genes for cytokines or growth factor inducing NO synthetase. Binding AGEP´s on neural receptors RAGE causes the induction of oxidative stress, protein kinase C and NFκB responsible for inflammatory processes and apoptosis of nerve cells. As vasa nervorum supply nerve cells, diabetic neuropathy is caused also by changes of endothelial cells.

2.2 Polyole pathway

Polyole pathway has physiologically role in reduction of toxic aldehydes arisen due to reactive oxygen species (ROS) into inactive alcohols. An initial and rate limiting enzyme of this pathway is aldose reductase which uses reduced form of nicotinamide adenine dinucleotide phosphate (NADPH) as a cofactor. Raising intracelular concentration of glucose increases the activity of this enzyme by which glucose is reduced into sorbitol and next into fructose. Elevated activity of aldose reductase leads to decrease of concentration of NADPH (needed also for glutathione reductase activity), by which intracelular oxidative stress is raising. Accumulation of osmotic active sorbitol and fructose causes the reduction of myoinositol and taurine in nerve fibers and decrement in membrane Na^+K^+ATP-ase activity. These processes lead to slow of axonal transport. Also oxidative stress and protein kinase C induce the sorbitol origin, apoptosis of nerve cells and microvascular dysfunction.

2.3 Oxidative stress

Biochemical and metabolic changes in diabetes duration cause the increase of reactive oxygen species (ROS) origin and also decrease of antioxidant systems activity. ROS, especially superoxid anion cause damage of endothelial cells leading to diabetic microangiopathy. In hyperglycemia condition endothelial cells are exposed to major glucose turnover, from glycolysis through pyruvate decarboxylasis into Krebs cycle with consequence of higher transport of electrones through mitochondrial enzymes. Electron-overloaded mitochondria produces significant amount of superoxid anions that lead into nitric oxid decrese, DNA damage, AGEP´s formation, protein kinase C activation and even polyole pathway activation.

Oxidative stress induces mRNA expression of tissue growth factor β1 (TGF- β1) and fibronectin playing important role in renal damage as they increase the extracellular matrix production. Overproduction of ROS alters the mesangial cells - the most important in diabetic nephropathy development - and supports the cell processes leading to apoptosis (Ha et al., 2008). ROS increase protein kinase C (PKC) activity in mesangial and glomerular cells and PKC stimulates the hyperproduction of ROS. These changes together with non-enzymatic glycation of proteins lead to kidney hyperperfusion, hyperfiltration, extracellular matrix cummulation, renal vessels vasoconstriction, reconstruction of renal structure and even nephrosclerosis.

Oxidative stress can directly damage neurocyte myelin, macromolecules and membranes of nerve cells and induces their apoptosis. Considering the blood supply of nerves through vasa nervorum, also dysfunction of endothelial cells contributes to diabetic neuropathy.

Microvasculature of retina consists of two types of cells - endothelial and pericytes. Early signs of diabetic retinopathy are characterized by dysfunction of pericytes and consequently by dysfunction of endothelial cells. Oxidative stress together with AGEP´s induce nuclear factor NFκB and apoptosis of pericytes and endothelial cells. They contribute to thickening of retinal basement membrane, formation of acellular capillaries or microaneurysmas. Pigment epithelium derived factor (PEDF), glycoprotein of protease inhibitors family, is extracellular part of retina and was found in vitreous and intraocular fluid. PEDF can inhibit the growth and migration of endothelial cells, has antiangiogenic activity, cytoprotective and also antioxidant effect. Oxidative stress causes the decrese in PEDF leading to dysfunction and apoptosis of pericytes. The stability of vascular integrity is provided by angiopoietin 1 (ang-1), while angiopoietin 2 (ang-2) is its natural antagonist which break the connection between pericytes and endothelium (Patel et al., 2005). Oxidative stress and ROS increase the ratio of ang-2 / ang-1 in pericytes whereby impair the stability of retinal cellular structure.

2.4 Protein kinase C

Protein kinase C (PKC) belongs to the family of kinases responsible for intracellular signalisation in the cardiovascular, immunologic or other systems. Till now, twelve isoforms of PKC have been characterized according to the structure and cofactor requirements. The activator of the most of PKC isoforms is diacylglycerol. De novo formation of diaclyglycerol is enhanced in higher concentration of intracellular glucose with the consequence of increase activity of isoforms PKC-β1 and PKC-δ. PKC can be activated also by some growth factors, superoxid (induced by hyperglycemia) and by AGEP´s. PKC mediated phosphorylation of substrate proteins triggers a cascade of pathophysiological responses. Isoforms PKC-β1 and 2 deteriorate the blood flow through retina and kidneys, increase the capillary leak, induce the production of extracellular matrix and activate many inflammatory cytokines what contribute to microvascular damage.

Formation of vascular endothelial growth factor (VEGF), a cytokine with major role in retinal leakage, angiogenic activity and neovascularisation, is at least partly PKC dependent. PKC activates the release of adhesion molecules, tissue growth factor β, endothelin-1 and fibronectin. PKC also increases leucocyte adhesion through upregulation of intracellular adhesion molecules leading to capillary leakage, occlusion and microthrombosis. PKC activation mediates inhibition of Na^+K^+ and Ca^{2+} ATP-ase activity contributing to reduction in membrane transporter activity and thus changes in nerve conduction, microcirculatory flow and capillary pressure (Casellini et al, 2007).

Described pathways (Ido et al., 1996) act not individually but in connected interactions (Figure 2).

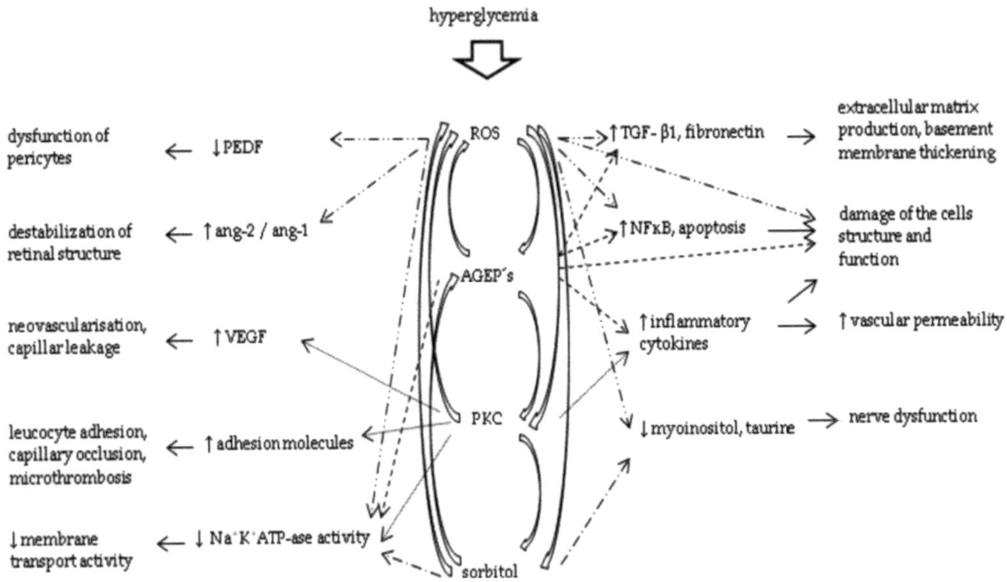

Fig. 2. Interaction between oxidative stress, non-enzymatic glycation, protein kinase C and polyole pathway and their impact on target structures (ROS=reactive oxygen species, AGEP´s=advanced glycation end products, PKC=protein kinase C, PEDF=pigment epithelium derived factor, ang=angiopoietin, VEGF=vascular endothelial growth factor, TGF=tissue growth factor, NFκB=nuclear factor κB)

2.5 Low C-peptide concentration

Disregarding hyperglycemia, the risk factor for microangiopathy development is decrease of C-peptide concentration in type 1 diabetes mellitus (Ekberg et al., 2007). C-peptide is producted by beta-cells of pancreas together with insulin and is used as a marker of endogenous insulin secretion as it is just minimally metabolized by the liver. The claims that it is biologically inactive molecule are now overcome. The binding of C-peptide to till now non-identified cell receptor leads to activation of G-proteins, increase of intracellular calcium concentration, increase of protein kinase C activity, MAP-kinase activity, increase of many transcriptional factors (NFκB, c-Fos), nuclear receptor PPARγ or antiapoptotic protein Bc12. On the cellular level, C-peptide improves nerve function and erythrocyte deformability by increase of Na^+K^+ATP-ase activity, improves the endothelial function and protects from microangiopathy by nitric oxide sythetase induction and has antithrombic effect by inhibition of adhesive molecules expression (P-selectine, ICAM1). It can inhibit the apoptosis by increasing the Bc12 concentration and can diminish the glomerular filtration by not completely understood mechanisms.

2.6 Angiotensin-converting enzyme

Angiotensin-converting enzyme (ACE) is circulating enzyme, exopeptidase, which participates in the renin-angiotensin-aldosterone system (RAAS) regulating the extracellular fluids volume and arterial vasoconstriction. ACE is secernated by endothelial cells of lungs and kidneys and catalyses the conversion of decapeptide angiotensin I into octapeptide angiotensin II (AngII) which acts like vasoconstrictor. ACE degrades vasodilator bradykinin and also other vasoactive peptides. Beside this, RAAS has a function in immune system - it regulates the extravasation and chemotactic migration of leucocytes, increases the expression of adhesive molecules, chemokines and chemokine receptors. T lymphocytes, macrophages and dendritic cells contribute to increase of renin and Ang II releasing through production of TNF and IL-1. According to the recent information, RAAS and Ang II have influence on origin of autoimmune diseases (Tippisetty et al., 2011). Ang II acts also like growth factor regulating the cell growth and tissue expansion what can lead to cell hyperthrophy and fibrotic changes of tissues.

2.7 Risk factors

An important role of diabetes *compensation* in development of chronic diabetic complications was proved by multicentric randomized study Diabetes Control and Complication Trial (DCCT) between 1983 and 1993 (DCCT Research Group, 1993). 1441 patients with DM type 1 (diabetes duration 1 - 15 years) were enrolled to the study, divided into two groups according to the treatment by either conventional or intensified insulin regimen. Children younger than 13 years did not participate but 195 adolescents were enrolled. The prevalence of micro- and also macrovascular complications was significantly less frequent in the group treated intensively compared to the conventionally treated group. The most of the patients consequently continued in the next study Epidemiology of Diabetes Interventions and Complications (EDIC) where all of the subjects underwent intensified insulin treatment. After 4 years of EDIC study, the prevalence of chronic complications was still higher in the group initially treated by conventional regimen despite actual good compensation. In the subgroup of adolescents, the intensified therapy led to decrease of the risk of retinopathy by 53%, neuropathy by 60% and microalbuminuria by 60%. In the next following of subjects in EDIC study, these differences were enhanced - patients treated from the beginning by intensified regimen had lower prevalence of retinopathy by 74% and of microalbuminury by 48% compared to the patients treated conventionally in the first phase. This study showed "the effect of metabolic memory" where each period of worsened compensation can negativelly influence the prognosis of the diabetic patient. Some studies with lower number of patients did not confirm the association between diabetes compensation and chronic complications (M. Javorka et al., 2005).

Diabetes *duration* is also suggested as an important risk factor for development of chronic complications. The significant correlation between diabetes duration and autonomic neuropathy (based on at least one pathologic result in two cardiovascular tests - heart rate variability, systolic blood pressure decrease in orthostasis) was confirmed in the biggest study focusing on chronic diabetic complications EURODIAB IDDM Complication Study (EURODIAB IDDM Complication study group, 1994) where 3250 patients with DM type 1 at the age 15 - 60 years took part. Similar correlation was not confirmed in some other studies (Scaramuzza et al., 1998) probably caused by different methods and lower amount of subjects.

Other risk factors were identified - increase in diastolic blood pressure ≥ 90 mmHg, increased triacylglycerides > 1,7 mmol/l, decrease of serum HDL cholesterol < 1,0 mmol/l, microalbuminuria > 20 µg/min, higher body mass index, presence of retinopathy, smoking and the period of puberty (Donaghue et al., 2009). The diabetes compensation in prepubertal period has lower impact on complication development compared to the period after gonadarche (Maguire et al., 2005). Many adolescents with DM type 1 have frequently worsened compensation due to endocrine changes in puberty leading to increase of insulin resistance (insulin like growth factor IGF-1, sexual hormones) (Court et al., 2008) but also due to excessive food intake, lack of physical activity, neglect of insulin treatment and hazardous behavior (alcohol, smoking, drugs, contraceptives).

Despite long lasting hyperglycemia, another important risk factor is *genetic predisposition* of the subject due to gene polymorphisms of enzymes involved in the pathogenesis of chronic complications origin and development (Donaghue et al., 2005). Probably other factors exist - immunologic, epigenetic, etc., which are not clear at present. This fact would clarify the clinical experience that some patients despite long diabetes duration and poor compensation do not have any signs of complications and on the other hand, some patients with adequate compensation and short diabetes duration suffer from some forms of complications.

3. Diagnostics

Diagnostic range of diabetic microangiopathic complications extends as it responds to ascending demands. Classic investigations (neurological examination, eye background investigation, microalbuminuria) could verify clinical manifesting forms of chronic complications. Nowadays, huge impact is put on the early diagnostics of clinically silent forms that has led to development of many new possibilities. New approach in diagnostics is investigation of gene polymorphisms of enzymes involved in the pathogenesis of microangiopathy that enables the individual approach to the patient and perhaps the "customized" therapy in the future.

3.1 Patient´s history and physical examination

Subclinical form of diabetic neuropathy is characterized as the absence of clinical manifestations of neuropathy, but specific tests can reveal the presence of some abnormalities. Clinical form can affect sensory-motor or autonomic nerve fibers. In **sensory-motor** form, the patient complains of sensory disturbance - paresthesia, dysesthesia, impaired vibration and / or thermal sensitivity, eventually of pain (neuropathic pain), and motor disturbances - decrease in muscle strength. Decreased tendon reflexes can be determined. These disorders can be expressed symmetrically or asymmetrically (Shy, 2007).

In **autonomic** form symptoms of disorder of various organ systems can be expressed:

- **cardiovascular** system: rest tachycardia, orthostatic hypotension, increased arrhythmogenesis of myocardium, cardiomyopathy, circulation instability, decreased tolerance of physical activity and heat, edema of lower limbs
- **gastrointestinal** system (Kycina et al., 2011): dysphagia, odynophagia, gastroparesis - nausea, diarrhea, constipation, fecal incontinence
- **urogenital** system: atonia of vesica urinaria, urine retention, common urinary tract infection, erectile dysfunction, painless while pressing testes
- **respiratory** system: decreased lung functions, prone to infections (Ďurdík et al., 2010), decreased cough reflex sensitivity
- **sudomotoric** system: feet anhidrosis, increased sweating of upper part of the body, sweating after food and at the night
- **endocrine** system: asymptomatic hypoglycemia, hormonal contraregulation disorder
- **other:** pupillary reflex disorder.

We note the patient's general condition, status and trophic skin and skin appendages - temperature, color, sweating, hair, skin appearance (the presence of dry, peeling skin), nail condition, pressure sores, infections. It is also necessary to assess trophic, tone and strength of selected muscle groups, loss of muscle mass, the state of the vascular system (pulsation of peripheral arteries) and condition of ligament structures of feet (shaped arch of the foot). Angiologic investigation - duplex Doppler ultrasound, transcutaneous measurement of oxygen saturation and blood pressure in lower limbs - is useful to detect the peripheral circulatory disorders.

Orientational neurologic instrumentary investigation involves (Consensus statement, 1988):

- **tactile sensitivity** investigated by 10 g Semmes-Weinsteins monofilaments which is attached to the top of the toe, 1st metatarsophalangeal joint, 5th metatarsophalangeal joint and the heel, bilaterally. Sensitivity is violated if a patient does not feel three or more touches of eight.
- **vibration sensitivity** investigated by graduated tuner (128 Hz). The tuner is attached to the thumb nail bed on the both legs. The tuner is graduated to 8 degrees, for damaged vibration sensitivity is considered the value of 3 or less at the age less than 50 years (the value 5 or less at the age over 50 years).
- **pain sensitivity** investigated by non-spiky sharp device on the tibia and feet
- **thermal sensitivity** investigated by glasses fulled by cold and hot water
- **tendon reflexes** (Achillary tendon, pattelary reflex) investigated by neurological hammer

According to the American Diabetes Association (ADA), the screening of diabetic neuropathy in adults is recommended to be done once a year by careful physical investigation involving examination of tactile, thermal, pain and vibration sensitivity and the examination of ankle reflexes. The combination of at least two tests reflects more than 87% sensitivity for neuropathy detection (Boulton et al., 2005).

Blood pressure. Measuring the blood pressure belongs to the basic investigations which can also reflect the diabetic nephropathy or cardiovascular disorders. It should be measured in calm, at least twice. Values more than 140/90 or more than the 90th percentile for certain age in children are regarded as hypertension and adequate therapy is set.

Eye examination by ophtalmologist including vision examination and eye background examination (color fundus photography or ophtalmoscopy) can detect manifesting forms of diabetic retinopathy. Slit lamp examination can investigate the spatial relations between retina and vitreous.

The recommendation of complication screening is presented in table 4.

	Recommendation of screening frequency	**Methods**	**Therapy**
Retinopathy	Once a year in children at the age > 11 years with DM duration > 2 years or at the age 9 years in children with DM duration ≥ 5 years	Ophtalmoscopy in mydriasis or photography of fundus	Improvement of DM compensation laser therapy
Nephropathy	Once a year in children at the age > 11 years with DM duration > 2 years or at the age 9 years in children with DM duration ≥ 5 years	Albumin concentration in the first morning urine portion or albumin / creatinin ratio	Improvement of DM compensation therapy by ACE inhibitors, decrease of BP
Neuropathy	Consensus was not achieved	History, physical examination	Improvement of DM compensation
Macrovascular complications	At the age 12 years	Serum lipids every 5 years, blood pressure once a year	Improvement of DM compensation, decrease of BP

Table 4. Recommendation for microangiopathy complications screening

3.2 Laboratory examinations

Advanced glycation end products (AGEP´s) are valuable markers for assessment of long-lasting hyperglycemia. In common practice **glycosylated hemoglobin** is used. Its concentration closely correlates with glycemia within last three months and it is influenced by many factors like recurrent hypoglycemia and processes influencing the life of erythrocytes (hemoglobinopathy, hyperbilirubinemia, uremia, hypertriacylglycerolemia and other).

Other AGEP´s - **N-carboxymethyl lysine**, N-carboxyalkyl lysine, pentosidine, methylglyoxal, imidasol - are used for evaluation of microangiopathy (Peppa et al., 2003). The parameter reflecting the glycemia during shorter period than glycosylated hemoglobin (because of its biological halftime) is **modificated albumin** – carbonyled albumin, carboxymethyl lysine albumin or glycosylated albumin. It is a marker of oxidative stress however further studies are necessary to confirm its importance as a predictor of chronic complications.

Other possibility for evaluation of diabetic complications are plasma markers reflecting the endothel dysfunction as they are released into the blood stream in relation to the endothelial damage (Adeghate et al., 2006), i.e. von Willebrandt factor, thrombomodulin, P-selectine, E-selectine, ICAM-1 (intracellular adhesive molecule), VCAM-1 (vascular cell adhesive molecule).

Diagnostics tests for diabetic nephropathy include urine sediment, protein urine test, **microalbuminuria**, urine and blood creatinine, blood urea and nitrogen. Microalbuminuria is usually set from 12-hour night urine sample while good glycemia compensation, normal blood pressure and without excessive physical activity. The result is considered as possitive when at least two from three urine samples investigated at the period 3 - 6 months with the one month distance interval are possitive. Investigation of metalloproteinase-9 in blood can detect earlier cases of kidney damage. Possible indicator of tubulopathy is **N-acetyl-beta-D-glucoseaminidase** (NAG). Its positivity in urine precedes the positivity of microalbuminuria in diabetic nephropathy. In the early stage, filtered albumin does not pass into the urine due to increased reabsorbtion in the proximal tubule and only NAG is present. Next, the reabsorbtion capacity of tubules is exceeded and microalbuminuria together with NAG is positive, in the advanced stages of nephropathy the positivity of NAG is caused by glomerular basement membrane damage as well as by tubular cells destruction. NAG is set as a ratio to creatinine in the urine (upper border is 0,25 U/mmol of creatinine).

3.3 Examination of autonomic nervous system

Cardiovascular system can be investigated by **heart rate variability** (HRV) by spectral and frequence analysis using the Ewing´s battery of cardiovascular tests (deep breathing test, orthostatic test, Valsalve maneuver) (K. Javorka et al., 2008; Havlíčeková & Jurko, 2005). The frequency of heart rate is not absolutelly regular but it oscillates about the average value. The result is heart rate variability which is influenced by autonomic nervous system - parasympathetic and sympathetic system together with endocrine system and other mechanisms.

In physiological condition HRV is significant as a consequence of cooperation of sympathetic and parasympathetic nerve fibers. In subclinical form of microangiopathy this balance is impaired and HRV is decreased. The first damaged non-myelisated nerve fibers in diabetic neuropathy is nervus vagus so rest tachycardia is a consequence of functional dominance of sympathicus (Maser & Lenhard, 2005). HRV is sensitive marker of heart rate regulation and activity of autonomic nervous system in adults, children and newborns (Havlíčeková et al., 2009). Heart rate variability is technically provided by computer system (VariaPulse TF4, Dimea Group, Olomouc, Czec republic) with telemetricaly scanning of R-R intervals by special software. The investigation is done in darken room, before noon, with avoiding of alcohol and smoking. Patient has loaded the monitorring belt around the chest to monitor the heart frequency which is telemetrically transferred into the computer. The subject is instructed (to lie, to stand up, again to lie, to make four deep breaths within 20 seconds) according to the actual test. The result is the protocol with parameters of high, low and very low frequency. The results are compared to refference values for certain age and sex (Tonhajzerova et al., 2002). To avoid false positive results is not available to investigate the patients with known disorders of cardiovascular and nervous system.

Other valuable method for early determination of microvascular complications is **cough reflex sensitivity** (CRS) (Čiljaková et al., 2009). Cough reflex is one of the defense mechanisms of respiratory system. The decreased cough reflex sensitivity is due to impaired nervus vagus function (as a part of reflex circle) and is detectable also in the first stages of microangiopathic complications (Behera et al., 1995). CRS is provided by inhalation of tussigenous matter in gradually increasing concentrations and is defined as the lowest concentration of tussigenous aerosol which provokes the cough. Two parameters are set: C2 as the lowest concentration of tussigen able to provoke the two coughs and C5 as the lowest tussigen concentration which provokes five and more coughs. As the tussigen capsaicin aerosol (hot pepper extract) is used, active in micromolar and izoosmolar concentration at pH 7,4. Capsaicin is diluted ex tempore in gradually increasing concentrations (0,61 - 1250 μmol/l). Aerosol is prepared by the nebuliser which is a part of Koko Pulmonary Function Testing. The subjects should breath through the mouth (with the clipped nose). The nebulisation is directed by the computer system and the aerosol penetrates into the respiratory system within 400 ms. The higher capsaicin concentration is needed for two or five coughs the more damaged is nervus vagus and the more developed is diabetic neuropathy. Each patient has done the spirometry before CRS. The investigation is contraindicated in patients who suffered from acute respiratory infection in last 4 weeks, in patients with allergy on capsaicin and relatively contraindicated in subjects with chronic respiratory diseases (bronchial asthma, cystic fibrosis). These conditions damage the defense mechanisms of respiratory system (cilliar epithel, mucocilliar transport), cause the higher sensitivity of respiratory tract to tussigen and so cause the higher cough reflex sensitivity. Mentioned conditions would cause the false negative results in the target to diagnose diabetic neuropathy. Four weeks are necessary to repair the respiratory defense functions after acute respiratory infection (Varechová et al., 2007).

Electrodermal activity (EDA) is simple non-invasive electrophysiologic method allowing to detect the changes in the ability of the skin to conduct the electric signals (Papanas et al., 2007). This skin ability depends on eccrine sweat glands activity which is regulated by cholinergic sympathetic nerve fibers and endocrine system through adrenalin concentration in the circulation. If sweat glands produce enough salt sweat, EDA examination detects lower electrical resistance and better electrical conductance. Subjects with diabetic neuropathy can have damaged also sympathetic nerve fibers leading to lower secretion of sweat. The decrease amount of sweat results in lower electrical conductance or higher resistance of the skin. EDA examination represents the sensitive method which can show the disorder of sweat gland acitivity and so is one of the possible method for diagnosis of neuropathy.

3.4 Examination of peripheral nervous system

Electrophysiologic examinations represent sensitive, exact and well reproducible methods for the diagnosis of neuropathy. The principle of **electromyographic** examination (EMG) is detection of action potentials arisen in muscle and nerve fibers. Commonly used is needle EMG and conductory examination of nerve fibers (Shabo et al., 2007). The most frequently examined are n.fibularis (motoric nerve), n. suralis (sensitive nerve), n.plantaris medialis and n.tibialis on lower extremities and n.medianus, n.ulnaris and n.radialis on upper extremities. **EMG** shows the muscle response to electric signal mediated by nerve fibers after injection of needle electrodes. Various action potentials, their shape, duration, number of phases and amplitude are evaluated while muscle contraction. The principle of **conductory** studies is irritation of peripheral nerve or nerve stem by electric impulses where the quality of nerve conduction (latention of response, velocity and amplitude) is evaluated. The dysfunction of nervous system results in decrease or even block of nervous conduction and decrease in the amplitude. The main advantage of EMG is the possibility to diagnose the subclinical form of diabetic neuropathy (Karsidag et al., 2005).

Quantitative examination of sensitive function represents the subjective diagnostic test based on patient´s indication. Unlike the clinical investigation of sensitivity, quantitatively exactly defined stimules are applied. The vibration sensitivity is evaluated by biotensiometer and by exactly defined vibration stimulus (Kincaid et al., 2007). Device CASE (computer assisted sensory examination) enables to determine the threshold of vibration, pain and thermal sensitivity. Standard test algorhitms are used and the results are compared to the refference values considering the localisation and kind of stimulus, sex, age and anthropologic parameters of the patient. The conductory threshold for three types of sensitive fibers (A beta, A delta and C) and pain threshold by superficial electric stimulation with 5, 250 and 2000 Hz frequency can be detected by new device Neurometer. The computerized system of randomly generated stimuli enables to define the accuracy of patient´s response.

3.5 Organ specific examinations

Several methods help to diagnose the diabetic gastrointestinal autonomic neuropathy, like esophagogastroscopy or gastrointestinal passage. Special endoscopic device enables to combine manometry and EMG signal registration in each parts of gastrointestinal system. New method is **electrogastrography** measuring the gastric myoelectrical activity from electrodes placed on the surface of epigastrium. In diabetic gastropathy, the normal electrical rhythm (3 cycles per minute) is replaced with bradygastria, tachygastria, mixed or nonspecific dysrhythmia (Koch, 2001). Gastric motility can be examined by ^{13}C octanoic acid breath test (Choi et al., 1997).

Diagnostic of diabetic urogenital neuropathy is possible by urodynamic examination, cytoscopy or ultrasound of urinal residuum. For the diagnosis of sudomotoric neuropathy colour skin tests with changing colours depending on sweat amount are available. QSART test (quantitative sudomotor axon reflex test) and TST test (thermoregulatory sweat test) are not available in common practice.

Respiratory complications (Brndiarová et al., 2011) of DM can be detected by lung function tests like spirometry, diffuse lung capacity for carbone monoxide or body plethysmography.

Examination of pupillary reflex latention is possible by classic investigation and also by **infrared reflex pupillography**. New non-invasive examination for early microangiopathy detection is **corneal confocal microscopy** which quantifies the pathology of small nerve fibers in cornea (Hossain et al., 2005). Cornea is the most dense innervated part of human body, contains A delta and C nerve fibers. Corneal confocal microskopy enables to analyse the density of corneal nerves, their morphology or branching.

Possible methods for diagnostics of diabetic retinopathy are **fluorescein angiography** showing retinal circulation, Amsler grid identifying what parts of visual field are damaged or eye ultrasonography used in the cases of vitreous hemorrhage or cataract. **Fluorophotometry** enables to measure posterior vitreous penetration ratio as the parameter reflecting the blood-retinal barrier permeability. New diagnostic tool for diabetic retinopathy and macular degeneration using LED technology is in development.

3.6 Gene polymorphisms detection

The new approach in diabetic microangiopathy diagnosis is establishment of gene polymorphisms for single enzymes which enables the individual approach to the patient.

Aldose reductase, rate-limiting enzyme of polyole patway, converts glucose into sorbitol in NADPH-depending reaction. Consequently, sorbitol is converted into fructose by enzyme sorbitol dehydrogenase using NAD^+ as a cofactor. In hyperglycemia condition glucose conversion by this way is increased leading to many metabolic and vascular abnormalities. Gene AKR1B1 for aldose reductase can appear in several variations which are associated with development of diabetic neuropathy, retinopathy and nephropathy. According to Donaghue et al. (Donaghue et al., 2005) genotype Z-2/Z-2 represented the predisposition to earlier development of neuropathy. Contrary, Z+2 allele was regarded as protective in relation with neuropathy development (Z=138bp in (CA)n repetitive sequence). Establishment of aldose reductase gene polymophisms in diabetic population could be important as aldose reductase inhibitors (epalrestat, fidarestat) have successfully been used the some studies. This is the first step to the "individually tailored therapy" when aldose reductase inhibitors could be taken in patients carrying genotype predisposing to diabetic neuropathy.

Uncoupling proteins (UCP1, 2, 3) are proteins in the inner mitochondrial membrane which are important in oxidative phosphorylation process, thermogenesis and also in protection against reactive oxygen and nitrogen species. UCP proteins reduce inner membrane potential through dispersion of protein gradient over mitochondrial membrane and so mitochondrial production of reactive oxygen species is decreased. G-866A polymorphisms in UCP 2 gene and C-55T polymorphism in UCP3 gene were associated with diminished risk of diabetic neuropathy development in diabetic patients (Rudolfsky et al., 2006).

Decreased activity of membrane pump **Na^+K^+ ATPase** plays significant role in microvascular, mainly in neuropathy pathogenesis. It is coded by several genes. ATP1 A1 is predominantly expressed in peripheral nerves and erythrocytes. Patients with type 1 diabetes who were the carriers of ATP1 A1 allele were more frequently affected by diabetic neuropathy (Vague et al., 1997). Identification of this risk factor can contribute to the prevention of neuropathy in the future.

Antioxidant enzymes are crucial in prevention against oxidative stress. **Glutathione-S-transpherase** (GST) represents huge family of GST isoenzymes which catalyze the conjugation of glutathione with electrophilic substrates resulting in less reactive and easily eliminated compounds. Substrates for this reaction are many carcinogens, drugs and also reactive oxygen species arisen in oxidative stress. The most intensively studied polymorphisms are genes of GST T1, GST M1 and P1. Null genotype of GST T1 and also null genotype of GST M1 significantly correlated with risk of coronal atherosclerosis (Manfredi et al., 2009). Deficit of GST as the result of null polymorphism of GST M1 and T1 was significantly related to the decreased heart rate variability which is a consequence of oxidative stress influence on autonomic nerve system (Probst-Hensch et al., 2008). Association between GST T1 and M1 polymorphisms with DM is not completely clear and differ according to the authors, region and population. Some studies claimed higher risk of DM 2 in GST T1 null and T1 null / M1 null genotype (Hori et al., 2007), according to another study, in contrary, the presence of GST M1 allele was risk factor for development of DM 1 and M1 null allele was regarded as a protective (Bekris et al., 2005). Some authors did not find any significant relation between GST polymorphisms and diabetic neuropathy (Zotova et al., 2004). GST T1 null genotype was associated with chronic kidney disease in diabetic as well as non-diabetic subjects disregarding GST M1 genotype (Datta et al., 2010). Similarly, GST M1 null genotype seemed to have no influence on end stage renal disease while GST T1 null genotype increased this risk in diabetic patients (Y. Yang et al., 2004). In young adults (average age 27) with DM1 was shown that GST M1 wild genotype represented a risk factor for diabetic retinopathy but not nephropathy. GST M1 null/T1 null combination did not increase the risk of microvascular complications (Hovnik et al., 2009).

Superoxide dismutase (SOD) catalyzes the conversion of superoxide into oxygen and hydrogen peroxide, which is split by catalase into water and oxygen. According to (El Masry et al., 2005), frequency of Ala/Ala genotype of Mn-SOD2 was significantly lower in patients with diabetic neuropathy and the genotype Val/Val was significantly higher in patients without neuropathy.

Hydrogene peroxide is harmful side product of many metabolic processes, so as the prevention from damage it has to be converted into less harmful substance. **Catalase** is enzyme localized in peroxisomes, functionally able to degrade the hydrogen peroxide into water and oxygen. In the study of C1167T marker of catalase gene has been shown, that C allele prevalence was more and T allele prevalence was less frequent in patients with diabetic neuropathy compared to the patients without neuropathy (Strokov et al., 2003). According to another study (Christiakov et al., 2006), 262 TT genotype of catalase gene was associated with higher activity of this enzyme in erythrocytes compared to the 262CC genotype. These results supposed protective effect of 262 TT allele against rapid neuropathy development.

Paraoxonase is a group of enzymes associated with HDL - cholesterol which plays role in hydrolysis of organophosphates and has also antioxidant potential. Three genotype forms of paraoxonases (PON) have been described till now. PON1 is synthesized in the liver and transported together with HDL into plasma. Its function is to prevent oxidation of LDL cholesterol. Inflammatory changes and LDL cholesterol serum level influence plasma concentration of PON1. PON2 is ubiquitously expressed enzyme which protects cells against oxidative damage. PON3 has different substrate specificity as PON1. Its concentration is not influenced by inflammatory factors and oxidized lipids. As PONs act in prevention of oxidized LDL formation and so in prevention of atherogenous plaques they reduce the risk of atherosclerosis and ischemic heart disease. 192 Gln/Arg polymorphism of PON1 presented the risk of myocardial infarction in young patients till 45 years while in 311 Ser/Cys PON2 polymorphism was not proved similar relation (Gluba et al., 2010). Association between DM and its complications with PON polymorphisms has not been found till now however decreased activity of this enzyme was described in patients with DM 1 as well as in patients with diabetic retinopathy compared to the healthy subjects (Ikeda et al., 1998).

The first and rate-limiting enzyme in myoinositol pathway is **myo-inositol oxygenase** (MIOX). Increased level of MIOX directly depends on increased glycemia and can be the cause of myo-inositol depletion in patients with diabetic complications. English authors studied single nucleotide polymophisms (SNP) in patients with DM type 1. These patients had decreased frequency of genotype combination CC (rs761745), GG (rs2232873) and GC (rs1055271) and less common haplotypes T/G/C and T/G/G compared to the healthy subjects (B. Yang, 2010).

I (insertion) / D (deletion) polymorphisms of **angiotensin-converting enzyme** (ACE) is characterized by presence (I) or deletion (D) of repeating sequency (287 bp) in introne 16. According to the combinations of alleles subjects with I/I, I/D and D/D ACE genotypes exist. Homozygotes D/D have nearly twice higher concentration of ACE compared to I/I homozygotes. Regarding ACE influence on capillary diameter, organ vascularisation and also inflammatory and autoimmune processes, ACE polymorphisms can effect also development of DM and its complications. Turkish authors claimed significantly more frequent prevalence of D/D ACE polymorphism in patients with DM type 2 compared to healthy subjects (Arzu Ergen et al., 2004). D/D genotype of ACE has been suggested to be in association with diabetic nephropathy in DM2 patients (Naresh et al., 2009). According to another study frequency of I allele was significantly higher in diabetic patients with polyneuropahty compared to diabetic patients without neuropathy. D allele was regarded as protective against neuropathy (Ito et al., 2002).

Determination of gene polymorphisms extends diagnostics of diabetic complications, enables individual approach to the therapy and gives the base for the "individually tailored therapy" in the future.

4. Management

Regarding the complex ethiopathogenesis, the management approach is also large. Till now, the only proved method how to slow the development of microangiopathic complications is maintain the optimal glycemia, even it is known that hyperglycemia is not the only one factor triggering the pathogenesis pathways. Arrangements contributing to euglycemia are also physical activity and adequate diet. As a supporting therapy, antioxidant alpha-lipoic acid is used although its effect was clearly proved just in intravenous application. L-carnitine and vitamins B have neuroprotective effect, vitamin C and E dispose of just poor antioxidant acitivity. Common possibility, expecially in adult patients, is symptomatic therapy like tricyclic antidepressants or pregabalin in diabetic neuropathy, ACE inhibitors in diabetic nephropathy, laser therapy in retinopathy. Another therapeutic options are in experimental line mostly proved in animal models, till now.

4.1 Euglycemia maintenance

Despite of various experimental and clinical studies, the therapy of microangiopathy remains insufficient. The only possible therapeutic approach which is concurrently clinicaly proved, is sufficient compensation of diabetes melltitus (Mokáň et al., 2009). The biggest study aimed at chronic diabetic complications, EURODIAB IDDM Complication Study, confirmed the significant correlation between glycosylation hemoglobin level and cardiovascular neuropathy. Even some authors denied this relation (M. Javorka et al., 2005), the optimal glycemia maintenance is strongly recommended as a prevention of diabetic complication origin. Children diabetic patients are treated by intensified insulin regimen. Patients with poor compensation are fully indicated to insulin pump therapy which best imitates the natural pancreatic secretion of insulin.

4.2 Dietary adjustment

Adequate physical activity and dietary style also attitude to euglycemia maintenance. Diabetic patients should avoid food with high content of sugar, food with higher concentration of fats and meals prepared by high temperature (fried, grilled) as these have excessive ammount of AGEP´s. Contrary, fruit, vegetable and boiled or steamed meals content lower concentration of these products. Prevention and treatment of diabetic nephropathy require also reducing salt intake at least less than 5-6 g per day. Advanced cases need restriction of phosphorus and potassium intake, as well. With advancing renal disease, protein compound should represent at the most of 20% of whole energy intake. Protein restriction of as much as 0.6 - 0.8 g/kg/day may retard the progression of nephropathy.

4.3 Symptomatic therapy

According to ADA recommendation (Boulton et al., 2005), painful form of diabetic neuropathy can be influenced by tricyclic antidepressives (e.g. amitryptilin 25 - 100 mg). However, the using of these drugs is limited in many patients because of anticholinergic and central side effects. From the group of anticonvulsives, gabapentin (1,8 g per day) and pregabalin are used (Rybka, 2007). Non-steroid antiphlogistics (ibuprofen, naproxen, indomethacin) are recommended only for short time due to their gastric side effects. The symptoms of diabetic autonomic neuropathy can be relieved by beta-blockers or ACE inhibitors. Other sympthomatic therapy is presented in table 5.

Symptoms	**Therapy**
Pain	Gabapentin, lamotrigin, pregabalin, temporary NSAID, magnetotherapy
Rest tachycardia	Cardioselective beta - blockers
Ortostatic hypotension	Sufficient ammount of fluids, bandage of lower extremities
Excessive sweating	Oxybutinin, glycolpyrolate
Gastroparesis, constipation	Prokinetics (metoclopramid, domperidon)
Diarrhoea	Probiotics, diet
Constipation	Lactulose, prokinetics
Urine residuum	Betanechol, doxazosin

Table 5. Symptomatic therapy of diabetic neuropathy

In the case of dyslipidemia, hypolipidemic drugs are used however we try to avoid them in the childhood. Every urinary tract infection should be treated and the prevention maintained.

Inhibitors of angiotensin-converting enzyme (ACE inhibitors) are drugs primarily used for treatment of hypertension and congestive heart failure. ACE inhibitors block the conversion of angiotensin I to angiotensin II. Therefore, they lower arteriolar resistance, increase venous capacity and decrease blood pressure, they increase cardiac output, lower renovascular resistance and lead to natriuresis. As the angiotensin II contributes also to ventricular remodeling and heart hypertrophy, ACE inhibitors prevent this effect. They cause the central enhancement of parasympathehic activity (Adigun et al., 2001) by which cardiac arrhythmia and sudden death are prevented. Angiotensin II induces several fibrogenic chemokines, namely transforming growth factor and monocyte chemoattractant protein-1 (MCP-1) which induces monocyte immigration and differentiation to macrophages augmenting extracellular matrix production and tubulointerstitial fibrosis (Amann et al., 2003). Thus ACE inhibitors can slow the progression of diabetic nephropahty. ACE inhibitors are superior to beta-blockers, diuretics, and calcium channel blockers in reducing urinary albumin excretion in normotensive and hypertensive type 1 and type 2 DM patients. Another possibility is represented by **angiotension II receptor blockers** which do not inhibit the breakdown of bradykinin and are thus just rarely associated with side effects like dry cough or angioedema. Although, hyperkaliemia remains as serious adverse effect so potassium monitoring is neccessary during the therapy.

Proliferative stages of diabetic retinopathy and some severe nonproliferative forms require **prompt surgical treatment**. **Focal laser treatment** (photocoagulation) can stop or slow the leakage of blood and fluid in the eye by laser burns of abnormal blood vessels. **Scatter laser treatment** (panretinal photocoagulation) can shrink and scar the abnormal blood vessels of the retina away from macula. **Cryocoagulation** represents additional operation to photocoagulation if this could not stop the development of prolipherative retinopathy. The treatment of macula edema involves focal laser treatment and intravitreal application of steroids (25mg triamcinolon). **Vitrectomy** can be used to remove blood from the vitreous or to remove scar tissue tugging on the retina. Surgery often slows or stops the progression of diabetic retinopathy but retinal damage and vision loss is possible.

4.4 Supporting therapy

Drugs with content of **alpha-lipoic acid** are used in diabetic patients with diabetic neuropathy (Ziegler, 2004). It is an antioxidant acting as a coenzyme of oxidative decarboxylation of alpha-ketoacids. It is easily transformed from oxidative form into reduced dihydroform what claims about its antioxidant potential. Metaanalysis of 1258 patients showed the improvement of neurological symptoms of diabetic neuropathy after intravenous treatment by alpha-lipoic acid (600 mg i.v. per day) (Ziegler et al., 2006). Unlike the intravenous therapy, the improvement of symptoms after peroral cure is not so clear. In 40 adolescents with DM, no significant decline of quantitative markers of oxidative stress, changes in glycosylated hemoglobin concentration nor in microalbuminuria was found after three months of peroral treatment by alpha-lipoic acid (Huang & Gitelman, 2008).

L-carnitine is common available nutritional supplement with function to transport fatty acids from cytoplasm into mitochondria thus help to utilise them. Its other role is antioxidant - to prevent the lipooxidation of fatty acids. In 34 of 51 children patients with DM type 1 (average age 12 years) was found diabetic neuropathy by nerve conductory examination. After two-months of treatment by L-carnitin (2 g / m^2 per day) the improvement of nerve conduction by 44% was claimed in subjects with early stage of diabetic neuropathy (Uzun et al., 2005).

Vitamins B are also used as an additional therapy. **Vitamin B6** (pyridoxamin) acts like carbonyl groups scavenger thereby diminishes the origin of AGEP´s. Benfothiamin is a derivate of thiamin (**vitamin B1**) soluble in fats with higher biological availability (Haupt et al., 2005). Thiamin and benfothiamin are cofactors of transketolase, an important enzyme of pentose-phosphate pathway, in which some products of glycolysis are degraded and so activation of metabolic pathways (AGEP´s formation, proteinkinase C formation) with tissue damage is prevented. Medicaments with content of **gama linoleic acid** (omega 6 unsaturated essential fatty acid), like evening primrose oil or borage oil, are appropriate as this acid is an important compound of membrane phospholipids and has anti-inflammatory, anti-thrombic and anti-atherogenous effect (Scott & King, 2004). **Vitamin C and E** as antioxidants act primarily non-enzymatic, can scavenge only part of oxidation stress end products, what explain their poor effect to prevent diabetic complications.

Vitamin D has an important role not only in calcium-phosphate metabolism but also in immune system and in renin inhibition (Agarwal, 2009). Patients with diabetes mellitus and especially with more advanced stages of diabetic nephropathy usually have lower levels of vitamin D and so are recommended to have supplementation of this vitamin. Vitamin D supplementation may reduce proteinuria in patients with diabetic nephropathy (deZeeuw et al., 2010).

Sulodexide is glycosaminoglycan with antithrombic activity containing two compounds - 80% of low molecular weight heparin and 20% of dermatan sulphate. Daily dose of 60mg (600 U) injected intramusculary during three weeks resulted in significant descrease of albuminuria and this effect lasted 3 - 6 weeks after drug withdrawal (Skrha et al., 1997). In the multicenter study, 237 diabetic patients with micro- or macroalbuminuria were treated by sulodexide 50mg per day for 6 months. Significant reduction of albuminuria was found similarly in type 1 and type 2 diabetes and was slightly greater in macroalbuminuric than in microalbuminuric patients (Blouza et al., 2010).

Calcium dobesilate is a venotonic drug with influence on membrane protocolagen, blood viscosity, aggregability of erythrocytes and trombocytes and with inhibitory function on PAF (Platelet Activating Factor). Some studies claimed that peroral treatment by calcium dobesilate (2 g daily for 2 years) improved the blood-retinal barrier permeability (Ribeiro et al., 2006), however randomised, double-blind, placebo-controlled, multicentre trial involving 635 patients with type 2 diabetes and mild-to-moderate non-proliferative retinopathy showed that treatment with calcium dobesilate 1500 mg daily within five years did not reduce the risk of development of clinically significant macular edema (Haritoglou et al., 2009).

4.5 Experimental possibilities

Ohter therapeutic possibilities are in the experimental line, till now. Many of medicaments effective in aminal models have not been applied in humans so their beneficial effect cannot be clearly proved. Huge negative of mentioned studies is lack of clinical verifying in children population.

Aminoguanidin is hydrazin derivative with its ability to bind reactive carbonyl compounds and so to prevent the formation of AGEP´s (Thornalley, 2003). It is available on Americal trade (75 mg tablets) as a nutritional supplement against aging and diabetic complications origin. According to double blind randomized study (Bolton et al., 2004) with 690 patients with diabetes type 1, aminoguanidin at the dose 150 - 300mg during 2 - 4 years had protective effect to diabetic nephropathy. Contrary, some studies do not claim its therapeutic activity (Birrell et al., 2000).

Alagebrium chlorid (ALT-711) splits kovalent bindings between proteins and glucose thereby helps to AGEP´s elimination (Little et al., 2005). Administration of alagebrium at the dose 210 mg per os daily in 62 patients with arterial hypertension led to the significantly increase in arterial flexibility compared to the group of patients treated by placebo (Kass et al., 2001). Peppa et al. (Peppa et al., 2006) gave alagebrium 1mg/kg daily to diabetic mice what had consequence in decrease the serum advanced glycation end products and microalbuminury. Also effect on diabetic nephropathy is assumed but further research is necessary to confirm it.

Recent studies showed beneficial effect of **C-peptide** substitution (Ekberg & Johansson, 2008). 46 adult subjects with diabetes mellitus type 1 and early stage of diabetic neuropathy enrolled the double-blind placebo-controlled study. Three months therapy by C-peptide (1,8mg per day) together with insulin substitution improved the functions of peripheral nervous system.

Inhibitors of aldose-reductase interfere directly into patophysiological process of sorbitol and fructose formation by polyole pathway. Epalrestat, ranirestat or fidarestat significantly improved the peripheral neuropathy in diabetic patients (Bril & Buchanan, 2006; Drel et al., 2008). According to the clinical study (Hotta et al., 2006) where 289 adult diabetics (type 1and 2) were treated by epalrestat (50 mg 3-times daily per os) within 3 years, the symptoms of diabetic neuropathy were significantly diminished compared to the 305 patients treated by placebo. The medicament is not available on common trade.

Ruboxistaurin, selective PKC- β inhibitor, can improve circulatory parameters of retina, can decrease macular edema, reduces microalbuminury and improves the symptoms of simpler form of diabetic neuropathy (Aiello et al., 2006). 20 adult patients with DM type 1 and 2 treated by ruboxistaurin (32mg per day) within 6 months significantly improved in symptoms of neuropathy compared to the 20 patients treated by placebo (Cassellini et al., 2007). In Japan, ruboxistaurin is farmaceutically produced for treatment of diabetic neuropathy, retinopathy and macular edema. In America and Europe it is used in the clinical studies, till now.

Apfel at al. (Apfel et al., 2000) found in their study that subcutaneous administration of recombinant human **neural growth factor** (NGF) during 48 weeks did not improve the nervous system function in diabetic patients. Hernander-Pedro et al. (Hernandez-Pedro et al., 2008) in the experimental conditions confirmed positive result after treatment by **all-trans retinoic acid** which stimulates the origin of NGF. An interesting study is also treatment by monosialic gangliosid GM1 which decreases the proinflammatory cytokines and increases the NGF in pancreatic cells by what extends their survival (Vieira et al., 2008).

Erythropoetin, initially identified as a hemopoetic factor, is also expressed in the nervous system and probably has neuroprotective effect. Chattopadhyay et al. (Chattopadhyay et al., 2005) deal with vectors gene transpher based on HSV (herpes simplex virus) which are originally replied in nervous fibers. They found that mice with induced diabetes had significantly enhanced the function of nervous system after HSV-mediated transpher of erythropoetin.

The using of angiotensin growth factor is controversial. Intramuscular gene transpher of VEGF (vascular endothelial growth factor) to the rats with induced diabetes caused the higher velocity by the nervous system compared to the control group (Schratzberger et al.,

2001). Contrary, VEGF induces angiogenesis and retina neovascularisation by what diabetic retinopathy is caused. Ranizumab and bevacizumab are monoclonal antibodies against VEGF. Several studies claimed their succesful using in patients with diabetic retinopathy and macular edema (Avery et al., 2006). The prospective trial evaluated the efficacy and safety of **intravitreal bevacizumab** in eyes with macular edema secondary to central retinal vein occlusion. Eyes were treated with 3 intravitreal injections of 1.25 mg at monthly intervals. After 18 months of follow-up, visual acuity was increased and central retinal thickness was decreased while no drug-related systemic or ocular side effects were observed (Zhang et al., 2011). The influence on diabetic neuropathy have not been described.

Neuropatic pain can be relieved by magnetotherapy. Weintraub et al. (Weintraub et al., 2003) proved significantly improvement of the pain after 3 - 4 months of wearing the magnetic lining in the shoes. Static magnetic field can penetrate to the 20 mm height and influence the nociceptors in the epidermis and dermis. 45 children at the age 5 - 17 years with diabetic neuropathy had significantly better velocity of nervous fibers after treatment by dynamic magnetic fields (Nikolaeva et al., 2008).

5. Conclusion

Diabetes mellitus is chronic disease with rising incidence where supraphysiologic concentration of hyperglycemia alters the biostructures in nuclear, cellular, tissue and organ level. Diabetes duration and compensation are not exclusive factors playing role in the etiopathogenesis of chronic diabetic complications. Recent studies have shown the impact of gene polymorphisms and have suggested the influence of other factors (epigenetic, immunologic). The fact that prevalence of microangiopathic complications increase with diabetes duration is undeniable but it is true in general not in individual view. Improvement of diabetes compensation is still the only known therapeutic possibility recommended to delay or prevent diabetic complications. However, some patients despite adequate compensation have some forms of complications and on the other hand, some subjects despite poor compensation and long diabetes duration do not suffer from any complications. Here, the importance of individual approach to each subject is shown as each one has the unique combination of gene polymorphisms predisposing or protecting him to diabetic complications origin. By this new knowledge, the advance from general to individual approach is possible. Huge hope with proceeding research is presented by new diagnostic and therapeutic options like "therapy to measure" according to the individual demand.

6. Acknowledgement

The work was supported by Center of Experimental and Clinical Respirology, CEKR II, co-financed from EU sources.

7. References

Adeghate, E.; Saadi, H.; Adem, A. & Obineche, E. (2006). *Diabetes Mellitus and Its Complications: Molecular Mechanisms, Epidemiology, and Clinical Medicine, The Annals of the New York Academy of Science Volume 1084* (1st edition). Wiley-Blackwell, ISBN: 978-1-57331-635-4, 300 pp., New York, USA

Adigun, AQ.; Asiyanbola, B. & Ajayi, A.A. (2001). Cardiac autonomic function in Blacks with congestive heart failure: vagomimetic action, alteration in sympathovagal balance, and the effect of ACE inhibition on central and peripheral vagal tone. *Cell Mol Biol (Noisy-le-grand,* Vol. 47, No. 6, (September 2001), pp. 1063-7, ISSN 0145-5680

Agarwal, R. (2009). Vitamin D, proteinuria, diabetic nephropathy, and progression of CKD. *Clin J Am Soc Nephrol,* Vol. 4, No. 9, (September 2009), pp. 1523-8, ISSN 1555-9041

Aiello, L.P.; Clermont, A.; Arora, V.; Davis, M.D.; Sheetz, M.J. & Bursell, S.E. (2006). Inhibition of PKC beta by oral administration of ruboxistaurin is well tolerated and ameliorates diabetes-induced retinal hemodynamic abnormalities in patients. *Invest Ophthalmol Vis Sci, Vol. 47, No. 1, (January* 2006), pp. 86–92, ISSN 0146-0404

Amann, B.; Tinzmann, R.; & Angelkort, B. (2003). ACE inhibitors improve diabetic nephropathy through suppression of renal MCP-1. *Diabetes Care,* Vol. 26, No. 8, (August 2003), pp. 2421-5, ISSN 0149-5992

Apfel, S.C.; Schwartz, S.; Adornato, B.T.; Freeman, R; Biton, V.; Rendell, M.; Vinik, A; Giuliani, M; Stevens, J.C.; Barbano, R. & Dyck, P.J. (2000). Efficacy and Safety of Recombinant Human Nerve Growth Factor in Patiens With Diabetic Polyneuropathy. A Randomized Control Trial. *JAMA,* Vol. 284, No. 17, (November 2000), pp. 2215-2221, ISSN 0098-7484

Arzu Ergen, H.; Hatemi, H.; Agachan, B.; Camlica, H. & Isbir, T. (2004). Angiotensin-I converting enzyme gene polymorphism in Turkish type 2 diabetic patients. *Exp Mol Med,* Vol. 36, No. 4, (August 2004), pp. 345-50, ISSN 1226-3613

Avery, R.L.; Pearlman, J.; Pieramici, D.J.; Rabena, M.D., Castellarin, A.A.; Nasir M.A; Giust, M.J.; Wendel, R. & Patel, A. (2006). Intravitreal bevacizumab (Avastin) in the treatment of proliferative diabetic retinopathy. *Ophthalmology,* Vol. 113, No. 10, (October 2006), pp. 1695-1705, ISSN 0161-6420

Behera, D.; Das, S.; Dash, R.J. & Jindal, S.K. (1995). Cough reflex treshold in diabetes mellitus with and without autonomic neuropathy. *Respiration,* Vol. 62, No. 5, (February 1995), pp. 263-8, ISSN 0025-7931

Bekris, L.M.; Stephard, C.; Peterson, M.; Hoehna, J.; Van Yserloo, B.; Rutledge, E.; Farin, F.; Kavanagh, T.J. & Lernmark, A. (2005). Glutathione-s-tranferase M1 and T1 polymorphisms and associations with type 1 diabetes age-at-onset. *Autoimmunity,* Vol. 38, No. 8, (December 2005), pp. 567 - 575, ISSN 0891-6934

Birrell, A.M.; Heffernan, S.J.; Ansselin, A.D.; McLennan, S.; Church D.K.; Gillin, A.G. & Yue, D.K. (2000). Functional and structural abnormalities in the nerve sof type I diabetic baboons: aminoguanidine treatment does not improve nerve function. *Diabetologia,* Vol. 43, No. 1, (January 2000), pp. 110-6, ISSN 0012-186X

Blouza, S.; Dakhli, S.; Abid, H.; Aissaoui, M.; Ardhaoui, I.; Ben Abdallah, N.; Ben Brahim, S.; Ben Ghorbel, I.; Ben Salem, N.; Beji, S.; Chamakhi, S.; Derbel, A.; Derouiche, F.; Djait, F.; Doghri, T.; Fourti, Y.; Gharbi, F.; Jellouli, K.; Jellazi, N.; Kamoun, K.; Khedher, A.; Letaief, A.; Limam, R.; Mekaouer, A.; Miledi, R.; Nagati, K.; Naouar, M.; Sellem, S.; Tarzi, H.; Turki, S.; Zidi, B. & Achour, A.; DAVET (Diabetic Albuminuria Vessel Tunisia Study Investigators). (2010). Efficacy of low-dose oral sulodexide in the management of diabetic nephropathy. *J Nephrol*, Vol. 23, No. 4, (July-August 2010), pp. 415-24, ISSN 1121-8428

Bolton, W.K.; Cattran, D.C.; Williams, M.E.; Adler, S.G.; Appel, G.B., Cartwright, K.; Foiles, P.G.; Freedman, B.I.; Raskin, P.; Ratner, R.E.; Spinowitz, B.S.; Whittier, F.C. & Wuerth, J.P.; ACTION I Investigator Group. (2004). Randomized trial of an inhibitor of formation of advenced glycation end products in diabetic nephropathy. *Am J Nephrol*, Vol. 24, No. 1, (January-February 2004), pp. 32-40, ISSN 0250-8095

Boulton, A.J.M.; Vinik, A.I.; Arezzo, J.C.; Bril, V.; Feldman, E.L.; Freeman, R.; Malik, R.A.; Maser, R.E.; Sosenko, J.M. & Ziegler, D. (2005). Diabetic Neuropathies. A statement by the American Diabetes Association. *Diabetes Care*, Vol. 28, No. 4, (April 2005), pp. 956 - 962, ISSN 0149-5992

Bril, V. & Buchanan, R.A. (2006). Long-term effects of ranirestat (AS-3201) on peripheral nerve function in patients with diabetic sensorimotor polyneuropathy. *Diabetes Care, Vol. 29, No. 1, (January* 2006), pp. 68–72, ISSN 0149-5992

Brndiarová, M.; Mikler, J.; Bánovčin, P.; Michnová, T. & Fábry, J. (2011). Extraesophageal reflux - otorhinolaryngological complication of gastroesophageal reflux. *Čes.-slov. Pediat*, Vol 66, No. 2, (February 2011), pp. 85 - 91, ISSN 1803-6597

Brownlee, M. (2005). The pathobiology of diabetic complications: a unifying mechanism. *Diabetes, Vol. 54, No. 6, (June* 2005), p. 1615–25, ISSN 0012-1797

Casellini, C.M.; Barlow, P.M.; Rice, A.L.; Casey, M.; Simmons, K.; Pittenger, G.; Bastyr, E.J.3rd; Wolka, A.M. & Vinik, A.I. (2007). A 6-month, randomized, double-masked, placebo-controlled study evaluating the effects of the protein kinase C-beta inhibitor ruboxistaurin on skin microvascular blood flow and other measures of diabetic peripheral neuropathy. *Diabetes Care*, Vol 30, No. 4, (April 2007), pp. 896-902, ISSN 0149-5992

Chattopadhyay, M.; Wolfe, D.P.; Krisky, D.M.;, Walter Cp:; Glorioso, J.C.; Mata, M. & Fink, D.J. (2005). Gene Therapy of Diabetic Neuropaty Using HSV-Mediated Transfer of Erythropoetin to Dorsal Root Ganglion In Vivo. *Molecular Therapy*, Vol. 11, Suppl. 1, (May 2005), pp. S249, ISSN 1525-0016

Christiakov, D.A.; Zotova, E.V.; Savosťanov, K.V.; Bursa, T.R.; Galeev, I.V.; Strokov, I.A. & Nosikov, V.V. (2006). The 262T>C promotor polymorhism of the catalase gene is associated with diabetic neuropathy in type 1 diabetic Russian patients. *Diabetes Metab*, Vol. 32, No. 1, (February 2006), pp. 63-8, ISSN 1262-3636

Choi, M.G.; Camilleri, M.; Burton, D.D.; Zinsmeister, A.R.; Forstrom, L.A. & Nair, K.S. (1997). 13C octanoic acid breath test for gastric emptying of solids: accuracy, reproducibility, and comparison with scintigraphy. *Gastroenterology*, Vol. 112, No. 4, (April 1997), pp. 1155-62, ISSN 0016-5085

Ciljakova, M.; Vojtkova, J.; Durdik, P.; Turcan, T.; Petrikova, M.; Michnova, Z. & Banovcin, P. (2009). Cough reflex sensitivity in adolescents with diabetic autonomic neuropathy. *Eur J Med Res*, Vol. 14, Suppl 4, (December 2009), pp. 45-8, ISSN 0949-2321

Consensus statement. (1988). Report and recommendations of the San Antonio Conference on Diabetic neuropathy: American Diabetes Association / American Academy of Neurology. *Diabetes Care*, Vol. 11, No. 7, (July 1988), pp. 592 - 98, ISSN 0149-5992

Court, J.M.; Cameron, F.J.; Berg-Kelly, K. & Swift, P.G.F. (2008). Diabetes in adolescence. *Pediatric Diabetes*, Vol. 9, No. 3, (June 2008), pp. 255 - 262, ISSN 1399-5448

Cvetković, T.; Mitić, B.; Lazarević, G.; Vlahović, P.; Antić, S. & Stefanovič. V. (2009). Oxidative stress parameters as possible urine markers in patients with diabetic nephropathy. *J Diabetes Complications*, Vol. 23, No. 5, (September - October 2009), pp. 337-42, ISSN 1056-8727

Datta, S.K.; Kumar, V.; Pathak, R.; Tripathi, A.K.; Ahmed, R.S.; Kalra, O.P. & Banerjee, B.D. (2010). Association of glutathione S-transferase M1 and T1 gene polymorphism with oxidative stress in diabetic and nondiabetic chronic kidney disease. *Ren Fail*, Vol. 32, No. 10, (2010), pp. 1189-95, ISSN 0886-022X

DCCT Research Group. (1993). The effect of intensive treatment of diabetes on the development and progression of long - term complications in insulin-dependent diabetes. *N Engl J Med*, Vol. 329, No. 14, (September 1993), pp. 977 - 986, ISSN 0028-4793

Donaghue, K.C.; Chiarelli, F.; Trotta, D.; Allgrove, J. & Dahl-Jorgensen, K. (2009). Microvascular and macrovascular complications associated with diabetes in children and adolescents. ISPAD Clinical Practice Consensus Guidelines 2009 Compendium. *Pediatric Diabetes*, Vol. 10, Suppl. 12, (September 2009), pp. 195 - 203, ISSN 1399-5448

Donaghue, K.C.; Margan, S.H.; Chan, A.K..; Holloway, B.; Silink, M.; Rangel, T. & Bennetts, B. (2005). The association of aldose reductase gene (AKR1B1) polymorphisms with diabetic neuropathy in adolescents. *Diabet Med*, Vol. 22, No. 10, (October 2005), pp. 1315-20, ISSN 0742-3071

Drel, V.R.; Pachem, P.; Ali, T.K.; Shin, J.; Julius, U.; El-Remessy, A.B. & Obrosova, I.G. (2008). Aldose reductase inhibitor fidarestat counteracts diabetes- associated cataract formation, retina oxidative- nitrosative stress, glial activation, and apoptosis. *Int J Mol Med*, Vol. 21, No. 6, (June 2008), pp. 667-676, ISSN 1107-3756

Ďurdík, P.; Fedor, M.; Jeseňák, M.; Hamžíková, J.; Knotková, H. & Bánovčin, P. (2010). Staphylococcus intermedius - rare pathogen of acute meningitis. *Int J Infect Dis*, Vol. 14, Suppl. 3, (September 2010), pp. e236 - e238, ISSN 1201-9712

Ekberg, K.; Brismar, T.; Johansson, BL.; Lindstrom, P.; Juntti-Berggren, L.; Norrby, A.; Berne, C.; Arnqvist, H.J.; Bolinder, J. & Wahren, J. (2007). C-Peptide replacement therapy and sensory nerve function in type 1 diabetic neuropathy. *Diabetes Care*, Vol. 30, No. 1 (January 2007), pp. 71-6, ISSN 0149-5992

Ekberg, K.. & Johansson, B.L. (2008). Effect of C-Peptide on Diabetic Neuropaty in Patients with Type 1 Diabetes. *Exp Diabetes Res*, Vol. 2008, No. 457912, (December 2008), pp. 5, ISSN 1687-5214

El Masry, T.M.; Abou Zahra, M.A.M.; El Tawil, M.M. & Khalifa, R.A. (2005). Manganese superoxide dismutase alanine to valine polymorphism and risk of neuropathy and nephropathy in Egyptian type 1 diabetic patients. *Rev Diabetic Stud*, Vol. 2, No. 2, (Summer 2005), pp. 70-74, ISSN 1613-6071

EURODIAB IDDM Complication study group. (1994). Microvascular and acute complications in IDDM patients: the EURODIAB IDDM Complication Study. *Diabetologia*, Vol. 37, No. 3, (March 1994), pp. 278 - 285, ISSN 1432-0428

Gluba, A.; Pietrucha, T.; Banach, M.; Piotrowski, G. & Rysz, J. (2010). The role of polymorphisms within paraoxonases (192 Gln/Arg in PON1 and 311 Ser/Cys in PON2) in the modulation of cardiovascular risk: a pilot study. *Angiology*, Vol. 61, No. 2, (February 2010), pp. 157 - 65, ISSN 0003-3197

Ha, H.; Hwang, I.A.; Park, J.H. & Lee, H.B. (2008). Role of reactive oxygen species in the pathogenesis of diabetic nephropathy. *Diabetes Res Clin Pract*, Vol. 82, Suppl. 1, (November 2008), pp. S42-5, ISSN 0168-8227

Haritoglou, C.; Gerss, J.; Sauerland, C.; Kampik, A. & Ulbig, M.W.; CALDIRET study group. (2009). Effect of calcium dobesilate on occurrence of diabetic macular oedema (CALDIRET study): randomised, double-blind, placebo-controlled, multicentre trial. *Lancet*, Vol 373, No. 9672, (April 2009), pp. 1364-71, ISSN 0140-6736

Haupt, E.; Ledermann, H. & Kopcke, W. (2005). Benfotiamine in the treatment of diabetic polyneuropathy - a three-week randomized, controlled pilot study (BEDIP study). *Int J Clin Pharmacol Ther, Vol. 43, No. 2, (February* 2005), pp. 71–7, ISSN 0946-1965

Havlicekova, Z. & Jurko, A. Jr. (2005). Heart rate variability changes in children after cardiac transplantation. *Bratisl Lek Listy*, Vol. 106, No. 4-5, (2005), pp. 168-70, ISSN 0006-9248

Havlíčeková, Z.; Tonhajzerová, I.; Jurko, A.; Jeseňák, M.; Ďurdík, P.; Nosáľ, S.; Zeleňák, K.; Antošová, M. & Bánovčin, P. (2009). Cardiac autonomic control in adolescents with primary hypertension. *Eur J Med Res*, Vol. 14, Suppl. 4, (December 2009), pp. 101 - 103, ISSN 0949-2321

Hernandez-Pedro, N.; Ordonez, G.; Ortiz-Plata, A.; Palencia-Hernandez, G.; Garcia-Ulloa, A.C.; Flores-Estrada, D.; Sotelo, J. & Arrieta, O. (2008). All-trans retinoic acid induces nerve regeneration and increases serum and nerve contents of neural growth factor in experimental diabetic neuropaty. *Transl Res*, Vol 152, No. 1, (July 2008), pp. 31-7, ISSN 1931-5244

Hori, M.; Oniki, K.; Ueda, K.; Goto, S.; Mihara, S.; Marubayashi, T. & Nakagawa, K. (2007). Combined glutathione-S-transferase T1 and M1 positive genotypes afford protection against type 2 diabetes in Japanese. *Pharmacogenomics*, Vol. 8, No. 10, (October 2007), pp. 1307 - 14, ISSN 1462-2416

Hossain, P.; Sachdev, A. & Malik, RA. (2005). Early detection of diabetic peripheral neuropathy with corneal confocal microscopy. *Lancet*, Vol. 366, No. 9494, (October 2005), pp. 1340-3, ISSN 0140-6736

Hotta, N.; Akanuma, Y.; Kawamori, R.; Matsuoka, K.; Oka, Y.; Shichiri, M.; Toyota, T.; Nakashima, M.; Yoshimura, I.; Sakamoto, N. & Shigeta, Y. (2006). Long-term clinical effects of epalrestat, an aldose reductase inhibitor, on diabetic peripheral neuropathy: the 3-year, multicenter, comparative Aldose Reductase Inhibitor-Diabetes Complications Trial. *Diabetes Care, Vol. 29, No. 7, (July* 2006), pp. 1538–44, ISSN 0149-5992

Hovnik, T.; Dolzan, V.; Bratina, N.U.; Podkrajsek, K.T. & Battelino, T. (2009). Genetic polymorphisms in genes encoding antioxidant enzymes are associated with diabetic retinopathy in type 1 diabetes. *Diabetes Care*, Vol. 32, No. 12, (December 2009), pp. 2258-62, ISSN 0149-5992

Huang, E.A. & Gitelman, S.E. (2008). The effect of oral alpha-lipoic acid on oxidative stress in adolescents with type 1 diabetes mellitus. *Pediatric Diabetes*, Vol. 9, No. 3pt2, (June 2008), pp. 69-73, ISSN 1399-5448

Ido, Y.; Kilo, C. & Williamson, J.R. (1996). Interactions between the sorbitol pathway, non-enzymatic glycation, and diabetic vascular dysfunction. *Nephrol Dial Transplant*, Vol. 11, Suppl. 5, (1996), pp. 72-5, ISSN 0931-0509

Ikeda, Y.; Suehiro, T.; Inoue, M.; Nakauchi, Y.; Morita, T.; Arii, K.; Ito, H.; Kumon, Y. & Hashimoto, K. (1998). Serum paraoxonase activity and its relationship to diabetic complications in patients with non-insulin-dependent diabetes mellitus. *Metabolism*, Vol 47, No. 5, (May 1998), pp. 598 - 602, ISSN 0026-0495

Ito, H.; Tsukui, S.; Kanda, T.; Utsugi, T.; Ohno, T. & Kurabayashi. M. (2002). Angiotensin-converting enzyme insertion/deletion polymorphism and polyneuropathy in type 2 diabetes without macroalbuminuria. *J Int Med Res*, Vol. 30, No. 5, (September-October 2002), pp. 476-82, ISSN 0300-0605

Javorka, K.; Javorka, M. & Javorková, J. (2008). Variabilita frekvencie srdca a diabetes mellitus. In: *Variabilita frekvencie srdca*, Javorka, K. (Ed.), pp. 124-133, Osveta, ISBN 978-80-8063-269-4, Martin, Slovakia

Javorka, M.; Javorková, J.; Tonhajzerová, I.; Calkovska, A. & Javorka, K. (2005). Heart rate variability in young patiens with diabetes mellitus and healthy subjects explored by Poincaré and sequence plots. *Clin Physiol Funct Imaging*, Vol. 25, No. 2, (March 2005), pp. 119-27, ISSN 1475-0961

Karsidag, S.; Morali, S.; Sargin, M.; Salman, S.; Karsidag, K. & Us, O. (2005). The electrophysiological findings of subclinical neuropathy in patients with recently diagnosed type 1 diabetes mellitus. *Diabetes Res Clin Pract*, Vol. 67, No. 3, (March 2005), pp. 211-9, ISSN 0168-8227

Kass, D.A.; Shapiro, E.P.; Kawaguchi, M.; Capriotti, A.R.; Scuteri, A.; deGroof, R.C. & Lakatta, E.G. (2001). Improved arterial compliance by a novel advanced glycation end-product crosslink breaker. *Circulation*, Vol. 104, No. 13, (September 2001), pp. 1464-70, ISSN 0009-7322

Kincaid, J.C.; Price, K.L.; Jimenez, M.C. & Skljarevski, V. (2007). Correlation of vibratory quantitative sensory testing and nerve conduction studies in patients with diabetes. *Muscle Nerve*, Vol. 36, No. 6, (December 2007), pp. 821-827, ISSN 1097-4598

Klenovicsová, K.; Saavedra, G.; Zumpe, C.; Somoza, V.; Birlouez-Aragon, I.; Kovacs, L. & Sebekova, K. (2008). Maillard Reaction Products in Infant Nutrition. *Čes.-slov. Pediat*, Vol. 63, No. 10, (2008), pp. 565-573, ISSN 1803-6597

Koch, K.L. (2001). Electrogastrography: physiological basis and clinical application in diabetic gastropathy. *Diabetes Technol Ther*, Vol. 3, No. 1, (Spring 2001), pp. 51-62, ISSN 1520-9156

Kycina, R.; Edwin, B.; Sutiak, L.; Strelka, L.; Szépe, P.; Mikolajcík, A.; Drgová, M.; Vojtko, M. & Mistuna, D. (2011). Laparoscopic distal pancreatectomy for neuroendocrine pancreatic tumors--initial experience. *Rozhl Chir*, Vol. 90, No. 3, (March 2011), pp. 200-6, ISSN 0035-9351

Little, W.C.; Zile, M.R.; Kitzman, D.W.; Hundley, W.G.; O'Brien, T.X. & Degroof, R.C. (2005). The effect of alagebrium chloride (ALT-711), a novel glucose cross-link breaker, in the treatment of elderly patients with diastolic heart failure. *J Card Fail, Vol. 11, No. 3, (April 2005), pp.* 191–5, ISSN 1071-9164

Maguire, A.; Chan, A.; Cusumano, J.; Hing, S.; Craig, M.; Silink, M.; Howard, N. & Donaghue, K. (2005). The case for biennial retinopathy screening in children and adolescents. *Diabetes Care*, Vol. 28, No. 3, (March 2005), pp. 509-513, ISSN 0149-5992

Manfredi, S.; Calvi, D.; Fiandra, M.; Botto, N.; Biagini, A. & Andreassi, M.G. (2009). Glutathione S-transferase T1- and M1- null genotypes and coronary artery disease risk in patients with Type 2 diabetes mellitus. *Pharmacogenomics*, Vol. 10, No. 1, (January 2009), pp. 29-34, ISSN 1462-2416

Maser, R.E. & Lenhard, M.J. Cardiovascular autonomic neuropathy due to diabetes mellitus: clinical manifestations, consequences, and treatment. *J Clin Endocrinol Metab*, Vol. 90, No. 10, (October 2005), pp. 5896-903, ISSN 1945-7197

Mokáň, M.; Martinka, E. & Galajda, P. (2009). *Diabetes mellitus a vybrané metabolické ochorenia.* Vydavateľstvo P+M 2009, p. 1003, ISBN 978-8096-971398, Turany, Slovakia

Naresh, V.V.; Reddy, A.L.; Sivaramakrishna, G.; Sharma, P.V.; Vardhan, R.V. & Kumar, V.S. (2009). Angiotensin converting enzyme gene polymorphism in type II diabetics with nephropathy. *Indian J Nephrol*, Vol. 19, No. 4, (October 2009), pp. 145-8, ISSN 0971-4065

Nikolaeva, N.V.; Bolotova, V.; Lukianov, V.F., Raigorodskii, I.M. & Tkacheva, E.N. (2008). Non-pharmacological treatment of microcirculation disturbance in children with diabetic polyneuropathy. *Zh Nevrol Psikhiatr Im S S Korsakova*, Vol. 108, No. 11, (2008), pp. 43 - 6, ISSN 1997-7298

Papanas, N.; Giassakis, G.; Papatheodorou, K.; Papazoglou, D.; Monastiriotis, C.; Chriskakidis, D.; Piperidou, H. & Maltezos, E. (2007). Senzitivity and specificity of a new indicator test (Neuropad) for the diagnosis of peripheral neuropathy in type 2 diabetes patients: a comparison with clinical examination and nerve conduction study. *J Diabetes Complications*, Vol. 21, No. 6, (November - December 2007), pp. 353 - 8, ISSN 1056-8727

Patel, J.I.; Hykin, P.G.; Gregor, Z.J.; Boulton, M. & Cree, I.A. (2005). Angiopoietin concentrations in diabetic retinopathy. *Br J Ophthalmol*, Vol. 89, No. 4, (April 2005), pp. 480 – 3, ISSN 0007-1161

Peppa, M.; Brem, H.; Cai, W.; Zhang, J.G.; Basgen, J.; Li, Z.; Vlassara, H. & Uribarri, J. (2006). Prevention and reversal of diabetic nephropathy in db/db mice treated with alagebrium (ALT-711). *Am J Nephrol*, Vol. 26, No. 5, (2006), pp. 430-6, ISSN 0250-8095

Peppa, M.; Uribarri, J. & Vlassara, H. (2003). Glucose, Advanced Glycation End Products, and Diabetes Complications: What is New and What Works. *Clinical Diabetes*, Vol. 21, No. 4, (October 2003), pp. 186-187, ISSN 0891-8929

Probst-Hensch, N.M.; Imboden, M.; Felber, D.D.; Barthelemy, J.C.; Ackermann-Liebrich, U.; Berger, W.; Gaspoz, J.M. & Schwartz, J. (2008). Glutathione S-transferase polymorphisms, passive smoking, obesity, and heart rate variability in nonsmokers. *Environ Health Perspect*, Vol. 116, No. 11, (November 2008), pp. 1494-9, ISSN 0091-6765

Ribeiro, M.L.; Seres, A.I.; Carneiro, A.M.; Stur, M.; Zourdani, A.; Caillon, P. & Cunha-Vaz, J.; DX-Retinopathy Study Group. (2006). Effect of calcium dobesilate on progression of early diabetic retinopathy: a randomised double-blind study. *Graefes Arch Clin Exp Ophthalmol*, Vol. 244, No. 12, (December 2006), pp. 1591-600, ISSN 0721-832X

Rudofsky, G. Jr.; Schroedter, A.; Schlotterer, A.; Voron'ko, O.E.; Schlimme, M.; Tafel, J.; Isermann, B.H.; Humpert, P.M.; Morcos, M.; Bierhaus, A.; Nawroth, P.P. & Hamann, A. (2006). Functional polymorphisms of UCP2 and UCP3 are associated with a reduced prevalence of diabetic neuropathy in patients with type 1 diabetes. *Diabetes Care*, Vol. 29, No. 1, (January 2006), pp. 89-94, ISSN 0149-5992

Rybka, J. (2007). *Diabetes mellitus – komplikace a přidružená onemocnění. Diagnostické a léčebné postupy.* Grada, 2007, p. 320,, ISBN 8024-7167-18, Praha, Czech Republic

Scaramuzza, A.; Salvucci, F.; Leuzzi, S.; Radaelli, A.; D´Annunzio, G.; Fratino, P.; Lorini, R. & Bernardi, L. (1998). Cardiovascular autonomic testing in adolescents with type 1 diabetes mellitus: an 18 month follow up study. *Clin Sci (Lond)*, Vol. 94, No. 6, (June 1998), pp. 615 - 621, ISSN 0143-5221

Schratzberger, P.; Walter, D.H.; Rittig, K.; Bahlmann, F.H.; Pola, R.; Curry, C.; Silver, M.; Krainin, J.G.; Weinberg, D.H.; Ropper, A.H. & Isner, J.M. (2001). Reversal of experimental diabetic neuropathy by VEGF gene transfer. *J Clin Invest*, Vol. 107, No. 9, (May 2001), pp. 1083-1092, ISSN 0021-9738

Scott, J.A. & King, G.L. (2004). Oxidative stress and antioxidant treatment in diabetes. *Ann N Y Acad Sci, Vol. 1031, (December 2004), pp.* 204–13, ISSN 0077-8923

Shabo, G.; Pasman, J.W.; van Alfen, N. & Willemsen, M.A. (2007). The spectrum of polyneuropathies in childhood detected with electromyography. *Pediatr Neurol*, Vol. 36, No. 6, (June 2007), pp. 393-6, ISSN 0887-8994

Shy, M.E. (2007). Peripheral neuropathies. In: Goldman L, Ausiello D, eds. *Cecil Medicine.* Saunders Elsevier; 2007, chap 446, ISBN 1416-0280-56, Philadelphia, USA

Skrha, J.; Perusicova, J.; Pontuch, P. & Oksa, A. (1997). Glycosaminoglycan sulodexide decreases albuminuria in diabetic patients. *Diabetes Res Clin Pract*, Vol. 38, No. 1, (October 1997), pp. 25 - 31, ISSN 0168-8227

Strokov, I.A.; Bursa, T.R.; Drepa, O.I.; Zotova, E.V.; Nosikov, V.V. & Ametov, A.S. (2003). Predisposing genetic factors for diabetic polyneuropathy in patients with type 1 diabetes: a population-based case-control study. *Acta Diabetol*, Vol. 40, Suppl 2, (December 2003), pp. 375-9, ISSN 0940-5429

Thornalley, P.J. (2003). Use of aminoguanidine (Pimagedine) to prevent the formation of advanced glycation endproducts. *Arch Biochem Biophys, Vol. 419, No. 1, (November 2003), pp.* 31–40, ISSN 0003-9861

Tippisetty, S.; Ishaq, M.; Komaravalli, P.L. & Jahan, P. (2011). Angiotensin converting enzyme (ACE) gene polymorphism in vitiligo: protective and predisposing effects of genotypes in disease susceptibility and progression. *Eur J Dermatol*, Vol. 21, No. 2, (March-April 2011), pp. 173-7, ISSN 1167-1122

Tonhajzerová, I.; Javorka, K.; Javorka, M. & Petrášková, M. (2002). Cardiovascular autonomic nervous system tests: reference values in young people (15-19 years) and influence of age and gender. Clin Physiol Funct Imaging, Vol. 22, No. 6, (November 2002), pp. 398-403, ISSN 1475-0961

Uzun, N.; Sarikava, S.; Uluduz, D. & Aydin, A. (2005). Peripheric and automatic neuropathy in children with type 1 diabetes mellitus: the effect of L-carnitine treatment on the peripheral and autonomic nervous system. *Electromyogr Clin Neurophysiol,* Vol. 45, No. 6, (September - October 2005), pp. 343 - 51, ISSN 0301-150X

Vague, P.; Dufayet, D.; Lamotte, M.F.; Mouchot, C. & Raccah, D. (1997). Genetic factors, Na K ATPase activity and neuropathy in diabetics. *Bull Acad Natl Med,* Vol. 181, No. 9, (December 1997), pp. 1811-21, ISSN 0001-4079

Varechová, S.; Ďurdík, P.; Červenková, V.; Čiljaková, M.; Bánovčin, P. st., & Hanáček, J. (2007). The influence of autonomic neuropathy on cough reflex sensitivity in children with diabetes mellitus type 1. *J Psysiol Pharmacol,* Vol. 58, Suppl. 2, (November 2007), pp. 705 - 15, ISSN 0867-5910

Vieira, K.P.; de Almeida e Silva Lima Zollner, A.R.; Malaguti, C., Viella, C.A. & de Lima Zollner, R. (2008). Ganglioside GM1 effects on the expression of nerve growth factor (NGF), Trk-A receptor, proinflammatory cytokines and on autoimmune diabetes onset in non-obese diabetic (NOD) mice. *Cytokine,* Vol. 42, No. 1, (April 2008), pp. 92-104, ISSN 1043-4666

Villeneuve, L.M. & Natarajan, R. (2010). The role of epigenetics in the pathology of diabetic complications. *Am J Physiol Renal Physiol,* Vol. 299, No. 1, (July 2010), pp. F14 - 25, ISSN 1522-1466

Weintraub, M.I.; Wolfe, G.I.; Barohn, R.A.; Cole, S.P.; Parry, G.J.; Hayat, G.; Cohen, J.A.; Page, J.C.; Bromberg, M.B. & Schwartz, S.L. ; Magnetic Research Group. (2003). Static magnetic field therapy for Symptomatic diabetic neuropathy: A Randomized, double-blind, placebo-controlled trial. *Arch Phys Med Rehabil,* Vol. 84, No. 5, (May 2003), pp. 736-746, ISSN 0003-9993

Yang, B.; Hodgkinson, A.; Millward, B.A. & Demaine, A.G. (2010). Polymorphisms of myo-inositol oxygenase gene are associated with Type 1 diabetes mellitus. *J Diabetes Complications,* Vol. 24, No. 6, (November - December 2010), pp. 404 - 8, ISSN 1056-8727

Yang, Y.; Kao, M.T.; Chang, C.C.; Chung, S.Y.; Chen, C.M.; Tsai, J.J.; & Chang, J.G. (2004). Glutathione S-transferase T1 deletion is a risk factor for developing end-stage renal disease in diabetic patients. *Int J Mol Med,* Vol. 14, No. 5, (November 2004), pp. 855-9, ISSN 1107-3756

de Zeeuw, D.; Agarwal, R.; Amdahl, M.; Audhya, P.; Coyne, D.; Garimella, T.; Parving, H.H. ; Prichett, Y. ; Remuzzi, G. ; Ritz, E. & Andress, D. Selective vitamin D receptor activation with paricalcitol for reduction of albuminuria in patients with type 2 diabetes (VITAL study): a randomised controlled trial. *Lancet, Vol. 376, No. 9752, (November 2010), pp.* 1543-51, ISSN 0140-6736

Ziegler, D. (2004). Thioctic acid for patients with symptomatic diabetic polyneuropathy: a critical review. *Treat Endocrinol,* Vol. 3, No. 3, (2004), pp. 173-89, ISSN 1175-6349

Ziegler, D.; Ametov, A. & Barinov, A. (2006). Oral treatment with alpha-lipoic acid improves symptomatic diabetic polyneuropathy. The SYDNEY 2 Trial. *Diabetes Care, Vol. 29, No. 11, (November 2006), pp.* 2365–70, ISSN 0149-5992

Zhang, H.; Liu, Z.L.; Sun, P. & Gu F. (2011). Intravitreal Bevacizumab for Treatment of Macular Edema Secondary to Central Retinal Vein Occlusion: Eighteen-Month Results of a Prospective Trial. *J Ocul Pharmacol Ther*, (August 2011), [Epub ahead of print], ISSN 1080-7683

Zotova, E.V.; Savostianov, K.V.; Christiakov, D.A.; Bursa, T.R.; Galeey, I.V.; Strokov, I.A. & Nosikov, V.V. (2004). Search for the association of polymorphic markers for genes coding for antioxidant defense enzymes, with development of diabetic polyneuropathies in patients with type 1 diabetes mellitus. *Mol Biol (Mosk)*, Vol. 38, No. 2, (March - April 2004), pp. 244-9, ISSN 0026-8984

Part 4

Thrombotic Microangiopathies: Perturbation of the VWF-ADAMTS13 Pathway

5

Von Willebrand Factor-Mediated Thrombotic Microangiopathies

Leonardo Di Gennaro, Stefano Lancellotti and Raimondo De Cristofaro*

Hemorrhagic and Thrombotic Diseases Service – Dpt. of Internal Medicine and Medical Specialties, Catholic University School of Medicine, Roma, Italy

1. Introduction

Microangiopathy is a term which describes a disease in the small blood vessels of the circulatory tree. Thrombotic Microangiopathy (TMA) was a term firstly introduced by Simmers in 1952 which combined several related disorders that are associated with thrombus formation in distinct organs [1]. In this group of rare diseases, the pathologic presentation is dominated by coagulation disturbances and endothelial cell injury resulting in swelling or detachment of the endothelial cell from the basement membrane, intraluminal aggregation of platelets and mechanical injury to red blood cells leading to thrombocytopenia and organ ischemia [2, 3] (see Table 1). These features are really common to various disorders, however Thrombotic Thrombocytopenic Purpura (TTP) and the Hemolytic-Uremic Syndrome (HUS), represent the major and more investigated forms whose pathogenesis has been clarified only in the last three decades [2-4]. Both TTP and HUS occur at a frequency of approximately 1-6 cases per one million people, may affect children and adults, and may each have several distinct subtypes with overlapping symptoms, but caused by differing pathophysiologic mechanisms [5].

Virtually all properties of the normal microvascular endothelium are altered in TMAs. Endothelial cells synthesize many substances involved in coagulation and fibrinolysis, including prostacyclin, nitric oxide (NO), thrombomodulin, tissue-type plasminogen activator inhibitor and von Willebrand factor (VWF) [2]. Leukocyte activation and complement consumption are also involved in TMAs pathogenesis [6, 7]. Particularly, an increase in vWF have been claimed to account for the loss of physiologic thrombo-resistance and for the consequent widespread platelet aggregation in vascular beds throughout the body, creating a cycle of vasoconstriction with platelet and fibrin deposition and further thrombus formation [3, 6-8].

In this chapter we will focus our attention particularly on von Willebrand factor (VWF)-mediated forms of TMAs.

2. Von Willebrand factor: A multitask protein

Von Willebrand factor (VWF) is an abundant plasma glycoprotein produced in all vascular endothelial cells [9] and megakaryocytes [10]. Mature VWF is a large multimeric protein

---

* Corresponding author

composed of a variable number of identical subunits, each consisting of 2050 amino acids residues.

Differential diagnosis	Relative incidence	Additional diagnostic clues and associated organ failure
Sepsis	60.2%	Positive blood coltures, leucopenia may be present due to hemophagocytosis phenomena, fever, purpuric lesions, signs of consumption coagulopathy
DIC	29%	Prolongation of PT and APTT, increase of d-dimer levels, decrease of natural anticoagulants, neurological and renal ischemias
Massive hemorrhage	8%	Low hemoglobin level, history of previous hemorrhage, prolongation of PT and APTT, tachycardia and/or cardiovascular instability
Thrombotic microangiopathies	0.8%	Coombs-negative hemolytic anemia, severe thrombocytopenia, schistocytes in peripheral blood smears, neurological and renal symptoms, fever, normality of blood coagulation assays
Heparin-induced-thrombocytopenia	1.4	Previous use of heparin, elevation of platelet count after discontinuation of heparin, arterial thrombosis with skin necrosis

Table 1. Thrombocytopenia and organ failure: differential diagnosis in some clinical settings

The VWF gene (VWF) is located at the tip of the short arm of human chromosome 12 (12p13.2), spans approximately 180 kb [11] and contains 52 exons. In addition to the VWF gene, a partial unprocessed VWF pseudogene is located on human chromosome 22q11.2 [12].

The primary translation product consists of 2813 amino acids, wich includes, in addition to the mature subunit, a signal peptide of 22 residues and a large propeptide of 741 residues [13]. This protein sequence consists of repeated domains or motifs that are shared with other proteins. These are arranged in the sequence: D1-D2-D'-D3-A1-A2-A3-D4-B1-B2-B3-C1-C2-CK. The protein is remarkably rich in cysteine, and in the secreted protein all these residues appear to be paired in disulfide bonds [14]. The mature subunit is extensively glycosylated with 12 N-linked and 10 O-linked oligosaccharides, and the propeptide has three more potential N-glycosylation sites. The N-linked oligosaccharides of VWF are unusual compared to those of other plasma glycoproteins because they contain ABO blood group oligosaccharides [15].

The preproVWF undergoes a maturation process in the rough endoplasmatic reticulum (RER) and in the Golgi complex. In the RER a monomer of proVWF (275 kDa) forms dimers via disulfide bonds at the carboxyl terminus, and it is known as "tail-to-tail" dimerisation [14, 16]. Instead, in the apparatus of Golgi dimers form multimers through an additional disulfide bond near the amino terminus of the mature subunit ("head-to-head" multimerisation), yielding multimers that may exceed 20 million Da in size. Additional modifications in the Golgi include the proteolytic removal of the large VWF propeptide, the completion of N-linked and O-linked glycosylation and sulfation of certain N-linked oligosaccharides.

In endothelial cells, up to 95% of VWF is secreted constitutively, whereas the remainder is stored in cytoplasmic granules called Weibel-Palade bodies that are specific for endothelium [17, 18]. Similar storage are found at the periphery of platelet α-granules [19]. VWF is released as unusually large multimers (UL-VWF), which can be up to approximately 20 000 kDa in size [20, 21] and are the most adhesive and reactive form of VWF. UL-VWF form string-like structures attached to the endothelial cell surface, perhaps through interaction with P-selectin [22].

Once secreted into the blood, multimers are subject to competing processes of clearance and of proteolysis by ADAMTS-13 (A Disintegrin-like And Metalloprotease with ThromboSpondin type 1 motif 13), a multidomain zinc metalloprotease that is remarkably specific for VWF [23-27]. VWF multimers are cleared with a half-life of 12–20 h [28, 29], by a mechanism that may not depend strongly on multimer size [30]. The molecules usually appear as tangled, condensed coils, but under fluid shear stress are extended, and UL-VWF strings are cleaved by ADAMTS-13 at the Tyr1605-Met1606 bond in the A2 domain [31] to generate the range of VWF multimer sizes that normally circulate in the blood.

Hemostasis depends on the balanced participation of VWF, and this balance reflects a competition between the biosynthesis of large VWF multimers and their degradation by the ADAMTS-13. Defects in the secretion, assembly or intravascular clearance of VWF can cause severe bleeding disorders. Conversely, inability to cleave the newly released UL-VWF multimers [32-34] owing to hereditary or acquired deficiency of plasma ADAMTS-13 activity may induce spontaneous VWF-dependent platelet adhesion and aggregation [35], leading to disseminated microvascular thrombosis as seen in patients with thrombotic thrombocytopenic purpura (TTP). So, mutations in VWF cause bleeding in VWD, and ADAMTS-13 deficiency can cause even more dramatic VWF-dependent thrombosis in TTP.

VWF is not an enzyme and, thus, has no catalytic activity. VWF serves as the primary adhesive link between platelets and the subendothelium, and it also carries and stabilizes coagulation factor VIII (FVIII) in the circulation. It performs its hemostatic functions through binding to other proteins, in particular to factor VIII, to platelet surface glycoproteins (GPIbα and integrin αIIbβ3), and to various subendothelial components, such as collagens, proteoglycans and glucosaminoglycans. Binding sites for several of these physiologically important ligands have been localized in the VWF subunit sequence. The binding of VWF to platelets appears to be regulated by its initial interaction with connective tissue, and also by shear stress in flowing blood. Under the effect of shear forces (>30 dyn/cm ^{2}), VWF unfolding occurs and the protein exhibits an extended chain conformation oriented in the general direction of the shear stress field . The stretched VWF conformation favors also a process of self aggregation, responsible for the formation of a spider web network, particularly efficient in trapping of flowing platelets [36-39]. Thus, the effect of shear stress on conformational changes in VWF shows a close structure-function relationship in VWF for platelet adhesion and thrombus formation in arterial circulation, where high shear stress is present.

VWF, beside its well known engagement in primary haemostasis, participates in other biological phenomena of particular relevance for the field of bacterial infection and leukocyte recruitment and extravasation. The induction of endovascular infections involves complex interactions between surface components on the invading organism and various host determinants. Staphylococcus aureus is a major pathogen in endovascular infections, such as infective endocarditis, suppurative thrombophlebitis, or vascular or heart valve prosthetic infection. Intravascular infection due to Staphylococcus aureus requires colonization of subendothelium requires both attachment and resistance to detachment under shear conditions. It was demonstrated that VWF binds to, and promotes the surface adhesion of S. aureus. Staphylococcal protein A (Spa) has been identified as a staphylococcal adhesin, especially for the high molecular weight VWF multimers [40].

The process of bacterial adhesion causes migration and activation of PMNs that secrete enzymes and ROS to eliminate the pathogens. VWF is an important player in hemostasis but has also been suggested to mediate inflammatory processes. Petri and colleagues [41] found that VWF strongly promotes the extravasation of leukocytes from blood vessels in a strictly platelet and GpIb dependent way.

Moreover, very recently, are emerging new functions of VWF, including a new link between hemostasis and angiogenesis [42]. Indeed, it was seen that the angiodysplasia can be associated with von Willebrand disease (VWD) [43, 44], these evidences confirm VWF as a protein with multiple vascular roles.

3. Thrombotic thrombocytopenic purpura (TTP)

Thrombotic thrombocytopenic purpura (TTP), also known as Moschcowitz syndrome,is a severe life-threatening syndrome mainly characterized by disseminated microthrombi that occlude terminal arterioles and capillaries in the microcirculation of multiple organs, most frequently of the brain [3, 7, 8, 45]. TTP is a rare condition with an incidence of about 4-6 per million people per year. The annual incidence of idiopathic TTP in western countries is approximately 4 per million. However, idiopathic TTP occurs more often in women and black/African-American people. Pregnant women and women in the postpartum period accounted for a notable portion (12-31%; about 1 each 25,000 pregnancies) of the cases in some studies. For this reason TTP predominantly affects female subjects between 10 and 40 years old [5, 6].

In 1924 Eli Moschcowitz reported the first case of TTP describing a healthy 16-year-old girl suddenly admitted to Mount Sinai Hospital because of weakness and pain of her arms, pallor, fever, few petechiae on her body, anemia, and leukocytosis. Four days later she developed left hemiparesis and facial paralysis, became comatose and died. An autopsy showed multiple thrombi in terminal arterioles and capillaries of the heart, brain, kidney, spleen, and liver [45].

Clinically TTP presented with a pentad of signs and symptoms: thrombocytopenia, haemolytic anemia, fever, neurologic abnormalities, and renal failure [46, 47]. An increased numbers of megakaryocytes in bone marrow, alterations of erythrocytes (schistocytes), and elevated serum levels of lactate dehydrogenase (LDH) are other important features [48, 49]. Clotting studies are usually normal. The typical fragmented red blood cells are probably produced as blood flows through turbulent areas of the microcirculation partially occluded by platelet aggregates. Therefore, the severity of these abnormalities reflects the extent of the microvascular aggregation of platelets and is responsible for microangiopathic haemolytic anemia. Serum levels of LDH are extremely elevated as a consequence of haemolysis and leakage from ischaemic or necrotic tissue cells [49]. Anemia is usually severe, hemoglobin levels less than 10 mg/dL being reported in 99% of subjects. Hyperbilirubinemia (mainly unconjugated), reticulocytosis, circulating free hemoglobin, and low or undetectable haptoglobin levels are additional aspecific indicators of the accelerated red cell disruption and production. Indeed, a negative Coombs test is needed to confirm the microangiopathic nature of the hemolysis [46, 47].

The two main types of TTP are inherited and acquired [50]. In most cases, TTP remains idiopathic, nevertheless several factors may play a role. These factors may include some diseases and conditions, such as pregnancy, postpartum period, cancer, HIV, infections, and autoimmune diseases; some medical procedures, such as surgery, total-body irradiation, and blood and marrow stem cell transplant and some drugs, such as chemotherapy, ticlopidine, clopidogrel, cyclosporine A, quinine and hormone therapy and estrogens [46-50].

Inherited TTP mainly affects newborns and children and is due to deficiencies in the activity of von Willebrand factor cleaving protease (ADAMTS-13), while acquired TTP is secondary to presence of auto-antibodies directed against ADAMTS-13 and mostly occurs in adults and older children [51]. In this latter form, IgG autoantibodies that inhibit plasma ADAMTS-13 activity can be detected in most of these patients, resulting in a transient, or intermittently recurrent, defect of immune regulation. The IgG subclass distribution identifies IgG4 as the most frequent subtype (90%), followed by IgG1 (52%), IgG2 (50%) and IgG3 (33%) [52]. IgG4 was identified alone and also in combination with other immunoglobulin subclasses. In addition, the hypothesis was proposed that the identification of IgG subclasses may provide a useful parameter to predict disease recurrence [52].

In 1982 Moake first found that patients with relapsing acquired or congenital TTP had circulating "unusually large" VWF multimers, while ultra-large VWF was absent from the plasma of healthy persons [33]. Moake proposed that these subjects lacked a VWF depolymerase, possibly a protease, that normally cleaved ultra-large VWF. Then this VWF-cleaving protease was purified, and named ADAMTS-13 because it belonged to the recently discovered "*a* *d*isintegrin-like *a*nd *m*etalloprotease with *t*hrombospondin repeats" family of metalloproteases (see paragraph above).

In patients with TTP, the systemic clumping of platelets mediated by unusually large multimers of VWF often results in platelet counts below 20,000/ μL during an acute episode. Ischemia of the brain is common, and renal dysfunction may also occur. However, a severe renal involvement in a patient with a diagnosis of TTP may be confused with HUS erasing clinical distinctions between these two disorders [45-50].

A rare form of TTP, called Upshaw-Schülman syndrome, is genetically inherited as a dysfunction of ADAMTS-13 [46]. In these forms of TTP, the deficiency is probably inherited as an autosomal recessive trait. It may appear initially in infancy or childhood and may recur as 'chronic relapsing TTP' episodes at about 3-week intervals. The absent or severely reduced plasma ADAMTS-13 activity in familial TTP is a consequence of homozygous (or double heterozygous) mutations in both of the ADAMTS-13 alleles located on chromosome 9q34 (frameshift and point mutations) [25]. Patients with this inherited ADAMTS-13 deficiency may be surprisingly asymptomatic, but may develop a severe and life-threatening in all those clinical situations with increased von Willebrand factor levels, such as infection or pregnancy. In these patients episodes of TTP are reversed or prevented by the infusion of platelet-poor fresh-frozen plasma, cryoprecipitate-poor plasma (cryosupernatant), or plasma that has been treated with a mixture of an organic solvent and detergent [53, 54]. The infusion about every 2-3 weeks of normal plasma into familial TTP patients lacking effective enzyme production/release prevents, or reduces the frequency of, TTP episodes.

Plasmapheresis is usually not required. The plasma half-life of infused ADAMTS-13 activity is about 2–4 days. Since a plasma level of only about 5% of ADAMTS 13 is sufficient to prevent or shorten episodes of TTP a gene therapy could induce lasting remissions in children with the chronic relapsing form of the disease [55].

In most patients with a diagnosis of TTP, ADAMTS 13 activity is 0 or lower than 5 percent of normal. Really, ADAMTS-13 deficiency may vary from 0 to 100% across several studies [2, 5, 6]. The cause of this variability may reflect differences in ADAMTS-13 assay methods. Moreover, patients with secondary TTP almost never have severe ADAMTS-13 deficiency. Thus, ADAMTS-13 deficiency more frequently identifies a large subset of patients with idiopathic TTP who suffer from VWF-dependent micro-vascular thrombosis.

Furthermore, essentially all patients with a prior history of severe ADAMTS-13 deficiency will have it again when they relapse with TTP, whether they had normal ADAMTS-13 levels at some other time during remission. Thus, ADAMTS-13 testing may help to distinguish the different mechanisms of TMA in complex clinical situations.

The mortality is almost 90% if untreated, but if treated, the mortality is reduced to 15% [6]. Adults and older children with acquired acute idiopathic thrombotic thrombocytopenic purpura require daily plasma exchange [5, 6]. Adults and some older children with acquired ADAMTS-13 autoantibody-mediated TTP require daily plasma exchange until remission.

Plasma exchange allows about 90 percent of these patients to survive an episode of thrombotic thrombocytopenic purpura, usually without permanent organ damage [54]. The plasma exchange has several beneficial effects such as removing fluid making it possible to substitute with a high volume of plasma to increase the ADAMTS 13 activity; another effect is to reduce the extent of cytokines and other pro-inflammatory factors that mayleado to VWF production and a further effect is to remove antibodies that are involved in the process.

Some patients with acquired acute idiopathic thrombotic thrombocytopenic purpura and high titers of antibodies against ADAMTS 13 do not respond to plasma exchange alone [54]. For patients with idiopathic TTP, ADAMTS-13 deficiency is a biomarker for a high risk of relapsing disease. In general, patients with idiopathic TTP usually respond to plasma exchange and those with secondary TTP do not. The value of plasma therapy was demonstrated conclusively in a randomized, prospective comparison of plasma infusion and plasma exchange for the treatment of adults with TTP. Survival at 6 months was 78% with plasma exchange and 63% with plasma infusion, a significant difference in favor of plasma exchange (P = .036) [54]. Because of this trial, standard treatment for TTP today includes plasma exchange at 40 to 60 mL/kg daily until the patient has a normal platelet count and a normal LDH, and any nonfocal neurologic deficits have resolved. If plasma exchange cannot be performed for some reason, patients may be treated instead with plasma infusion at up to 30 mL/kg daily, provided they can tolerate the fluid load.

It may be possible to interfere with autoantibody production through treatment with glucocorticoids or splenectomy [56] Rituximab, the monoclonal antibody against CD20 on B-lymphocytes, represent another important possible strategy in these patient [57-59].

In this setting, rituximab appears to be effective at normalizing ADAMTS-13 levels and inducing durable remissions. Published small series and case reports have described approximately 100 patients with refractory or relapsing idiopathic TTP treated with rituximab, usually at doses of 375 mg/m^2 weekly for an average of 4 doses. Approximately 95% of reported patients have had a complete clinical and laboratory responses within 1 to 3 weeks of starting treatment, including a normal ADAMTS-13 level and disappearance of anti-ADAMTS-13 antibodies [58, 60]. However, secondary infections and side effects should cause caution in the use of rituximab. This has caused FDA to stop an ongoing randomized study, the STAR-study, in the US due to serious adverse events in the rituximab arm [61].

Mild acute reactions to rituximab infusions were controlled by premedication with steroids, antihistamines, and analgesics.

Relapses have been infrequent, occurring in approximately 10% of patients after intervals of 9 months to 4 years. These reports have all the limitations and potential biases of case series, and they should be interpreted cautiously. In particular, judging the efficacy of rituximab is difficult because patients usually receive multiple different treatments. Nevertheless, rituximab seems to rescue most patients with refractory or relapsing idiopathic TTP. Moreover, by abolishing autoantibody production, adjuvant rituximab at first diagnosis (combined with plasma exchange) might further improve outcomes by shortening the duration of plasma exchange, reducing early mortality, and preventing relapses.

ADAMTS-13 has been partially purified and produced in recombinant active form for possible eventual therapeutic use [5, 6]. Because plasma ADAMTS-13 levels of only about 5% is often sufficient to prevent or truncate TTP episodes, gene therapy may eventually extend remissions in familial TTP patients. Another possible new therapy is the infusion of an oligonucleotide aptamer designed to block the adhesion of platelet GP1ba receptors to A1 domains in the VWF monomeric subunits of VWF strings.

In the absence of life-threatening hemorrhage or intracranial bleeding, it is prudent to avoid platelet transfusions, which can exacerbate microvascular thrombosis. Aspirin may provoke hemorrhagic complications in patients with severe thrombocytopenia. Currently, according to main guidelines, an adult patient who has a suspected acquired syndrome that could be either thrombotic thrombocytopenic purpura or the hemolytic–uremic syndrome should be presumed to have thrombotic thrombocytopenic purpura, and plasma exchange should be initiated as soon as possible.

4. Haemolitic uremic syndrome (HUS)

Besides TTP, endothelial cells can be stimulated to secrete long VWF strings by inflammatory cytokines: tumour necrosis factor-alpha, interleukin (IL)-8 and IL-6, bacterial-produced toxins and oestrogen [2-7]. Therefore all those diseases or clinical conditions that contribute to this pathway could be responsible for a VWF mediated TMAs or predispose to this disorder.

Also HUS is characterized by low platelet count and microangiopathic hemolytic anemia due to platelet-fibrin thrombi occluding predominantly the renal circulation [4, 62, 63]. The most common of HUS, so-called typical HUS, affects about 70-80% of all HUS cases, mainly children and occurs in 9 to 30 percent of infected children about a week after an episode of bloody diarrhea caused by enterohaemorrhagic gram-negative Escherichia coli that produce Shiga toxin (e.g., Escherichia coli of serotype 0157:H7) [63]. This bacteria is found in manure, water troughs, and other places in farms, which may explain the increased risk of infection observed in people living in rural areas. The microorganism is transmitted to humans by food and water, directly from person to person and occasionally through occupational exposure. Fruits and vegetables may be contaminated and have been implicated in several outbreaks. Water-borne outbreaks have occurred as a result of drinking and swimming in unchlorinated water. Person-to-person transmission has been reported in daycare and chronic-care facilities [64, 65].

Also Schigella dysenteriae type 1 can be responsible for a toxin involved in typical HUS. Finally, rare, familial types of HUS may be caused by deficient quantity or defective function of a regulatory protein in the alternative complement pathway; or, more rarely, by defective intracellular cobalamin reduction/cofactor function.

As in TTP, in typical HUS large multimers of von Willebrand factor can be produced by endothelial cells due to E.coli Shiga toxin1 production. This toxin stimulates the rapid and profuse secretion of long VWF multimeric strings from endothelial cells, including glomerular microvascular endothelial cells. The initial and progressive platelet adhesion to long VWF strings may explain the glomerular microvascular occlusion and acute renal failure.

However, unlike TTP, HUS is not usually associated with the absence or severe reduction of plasma ADAMTS 13 activity. On the contrary, atypical HUS (aHUS), identified in about 10-15% of patients, affecting more often adults, has genetic causes and is frequently associated with gene mutations of complement regulators or components that form the alternative pathway convertase C3bBb, but is not a VWF mediated TMA. Childhood Shiga toxin-*E. coli*-associated HUS usually recovers spontaneously and does not require plasma therapy [66, 67].

5. Other secondary VWF-mediated TMAs

There are many secondary causes of TMAs; many of them could mimic TTP or HUS.

More recent data indicate that low or zero ADAMTS 13 activity is not confined to TTP and can even be found in a number of diseases associated with an increased tendency to thrombosis. Plasma ADAMTS-13 activity is often reduced below normal in liver disease, disseminated malignancies, chronic metabolic and inflammatory conditions, pregnancy and newborns [5, 6]. With the exception of the occasional peri-partum women who develop overt TTP, the ADAMTS-13 activity in these conditions is not reduced to the extremely low values (i.e., <5-10% of normal) found in patients with familial or acquired autoantibody mediated TTP.

Moreover, HUS/TTP form complicates immune diseases, in particular systemic lupus erythematosus, and increasingly is reported in association with the antiphospholipid syndrome [6].

Indeed, von Willebrand factor's susceptibility to fragmentation increases in response to rising levels of shear stress, which induces protein unfolding and makes vWF proteolytic cleavage sites more accessible to ADAMTS-13. It is speculated that enhanced shear stress in the severely narrowed damaged microvessels accounts for the abnormal vWF fragmentation observed during an acute inflammation. Evidence of increased capacity of fragmented vWF to bind receptors on activated platelets suggests that shear stress-induced vWF fragmentation may contribute to maintain and further spread microvascular thrombosis. In addition, or alternatively, the accentuated secretion of long VWF multimeric strings by endothelial cells stimulated by oestrogen or inflammatory cytokines may be required to provoke TMAs in some patients with very low plasma ADAMTS-13 values.

Plasmapheresis should always be attempted in secondary TMAs even though the efficacy has to be demonstrated.

6. TMAS associated to drugs

Cyclosporine, a cyclic nonapeptide, and tacrolimus, a macrolide, inhibit protein phosphatase 2B (calcineurin) in immune and endothelial cells. Cyclosporine- or tacrolimus-treated endothelial cells secrete long VWF multimeric strings. The latter process may slowly overwhelm the capacity of ADAMTS-13 to defend the microvasculature against platelet thrombotic occlusion and thrombotic

Microangiopathy [57, 59, 68]. There are some analogies with the pathophysiology both of diarrhoea-associated HUS and of sepsis/disseminated intravascular coagulation (DIC)/renal failure. In sepsis/DIC/renal failure, there is cytokine-stimulated VWF string secretion from stimulated endothelial cells associated with the partial consumption of plasma ADAMTS-13. Treatment for transplantation-immunosuppression-induced or chemotherapy–radiotherapy associated thrombotic microangiopathy is, to date, limited to supportive care and the discontinuation of any putative offending drug.

Ticlopidine and clopidogrel have been associated with the development of HUS/TTP, but this event is rare (1 in 1600 patients treated with ticlopidine after cardiac stenting). These drugs are structurally related derivatives of thienopyridine and act by blocking an adenosine diphosphate-binding site on platelets, which inhibits the expression of the glycoprotein IIb/IIIa receptor in the high-affinity configuration that binds fibrinogen and large VWF multimers.

Why these two drugs cause TTP is not fully clear, but of great interest, as patients with ticlopidine- or clopidogrel-associated TTP have a deficiency of VWF-cleaving protease activity in plasma that appears quite comparable to the deficiency observed in idiopathic TTP [69-71]. Probably, these drugs, such as quinine, should be associated with development of antibodies against ADAMTS 13 and in these patients plasma exchange is indicated [69, 71, 72].

7. The role of VWF in other arterial thrombotic diseases

It has been suggested that VWF plays an important role in the pathogenesis of arterial thrombotic disorders. Previous studies have shown the relevance of platelets and VWF in the initiation of atherosclerotic plaque formation. Both inactivation of VWF and inhibition of

VWF-GP1b interaction delay the formation of fatty streaks VWF. From a biological standpoint, it is likely that VWF contributes to the pathogenesis of early atherosclerotic lesions. Hence, many studies have investigated the association between VWF plasma levels and the subsequent risk of cardiovascular disease. In the ARIC study, the relative risk (RR) for coronary artery disease (CHD) for the highest vs. the lowest tertiles of VWF levels was approximately 1.3 [73, 74]. Moreover, VWF was found to play a relevant role in thrombotic microangiopathies occurring in diabetes mellitus [75]. More recently, compelling evidence has emerged about the association of high VWF levels with occurrence of ischemic stroke, particularly in the cardioembolic and cryptogenetic subtypes [76, 77]. On the basis of the known association between micro- and macroangiopathy in the brain circulation [78], we can speculate that high levels of VWF may contribute to the development of cerebral micrangiopathies, responsible for pathological lesions such as lipohyalinosis and fribrohyalinosis [79] that may evolve toward various types of ischemic stroke [77].

8. Prospectives and future directions

TMA is the result of various etiological causes and pathologic reactions with various clinical entities. Fortunatelly, TMAs are a rare group of disorders and number of patients invoved is usually too low to sustain an adequately powered study to compare different diagnostic and treatment stategies. Certainly, it is important to focus on a thorough history including the family history when deciding on a diagnostics. Particularly in TTP several promising multicenter trials are in progress and prospective observational studies and multicentric registries are enrolling adult and pediatric patients for longitudinal measurements of ADAMTS-13 activity, antigen, and autoantibodies, and ADAMTS-13 gene sequencing, for evaluating different treatments such as rituximab plus plasma exchange. These trials will address whether rituximab is best used as adjuvant or salvage therapy [80]. Because severe ADAMTS-13 deficiency will not be required for participation, this trial will include some patients with idiopathic TTP who do not have severe ADAMTS-13 deficiency, and the results should indicate whether such patients differ fundamentally from those with severe ADAMTS-13 deficiency in their response to plasma exchange, incidence of relapse, and response to rituximab. Moreover, these trials should clearly demonstrate whether rapid ADAMTS-13 assays could be useful for diagnosis or to guide therapy. Furthermore, ADAMTS-13 deficiency is not responsible for all cases of TMAs, and all the reserchers should look forward to recognizing and characterizing other causes, leading to understanding underlying unknown pathophysiologic mechanisms. At the moment, analysis of ADAMTS-13 and ADAMTS-13-antibodies may help to decide about continued therapy.

9. Acknowledgments

Financial support from Ministry of University and Scientific Research of Italy and Catholic University School of Medicine (Grant "Linea D1 - Anno 2010) is gratefully acknowledged.

10. References

[1] Symmers, W.S., *Thrombotic microangiopathic haemolytic anaemia (thrombotic microangiopathy)*. Br Med J, 1952. 2(4790): p. 897-903.

[2] Caprioli, J., G. Remuzzi, and M. Noris, *Thrombotic microangiopathies: from animal models to human disease and cure.* Contrib Nephrol, 2011. 169: p. 337-50.

[3] Moake, J.L., *Thrombotic microangiopathies.* N Engl J Med, 2002. 347(8): p. 589-600.

[4] Noris, M. and G. Remuzzi, *Atypical hemolytic-uremic syndrome.* N Engl J Med, 2009. 361(17): p. 1676-87.

[5] Zipfel, P.F., S. Heinen, and C. Skerka, *Thrombotic microangiopathies: new insights and new challenges.* Curr Opin Nephrol Hypertens, 2010. 19(4): p. 372-8.

[6] Mortzell, M., et al., *Thrombotic microangiopathy.* Transfus Apher Sci, 2011.

[7] Ruggenenti, P., M. Noris, and G. Remuzzi, *Thrombotic microangiopathy, hemolytic uremic syndrome, and thrombotic thrombocytopenic purpura.* Kidney Int, 2001. 60(3): p. 831-46.

[8] Byrnes, J.J. and J.L. Moake, *Thrombotic thrombocytopenic purpura and the haemolytic-uraemic syndrome: evolving concepts of pathogenesis and therapy.* Clin Haematol, 1986. 15(2): p. 413-42.

[9] Jaffe, E.A., L.W. Hoyer, and R.L. Nachman, *Synthesis of von Willebrand factor by cultured human endothelial cells.* Proc Natl Acad Sci U S A, 1974. 71(5): p. 1906-9.

[10] Nachman, R., R. Levine, and E.A. Jaffe, *Synthesis of factor VIII antigen by cultured guinea pig megakaryocytes.* J Clin Invest, 1977. 60(4): p. 914-21.

[11] Mancuso, D.J., et al., *Structure of the gene for human von Willebrand factor.* J Biol Chem, 1989. 264(33): p. 19514-27.

[12] Patracchini, P., et al., *Sublocalization of von Willebrand factor pseudogene to 22q11.22-q11.23 by in situ hybridization in a 46,X,t(X;22)(pter;q11.21) translocation.* Hum Genet, 1989. 83(3): p. 264-6.

[13] Wagner, D.D. and V.J. Marder, *Biosynthesis of von Willebrand protein by human endothelial cells. Identification of a large precursor polypeptide chain.* J Biol Chem, 1983. 258(4): p. 2065-7.

[14] Marti, T., et al., *Identification of disulfide-bridged substructures within human von Willebrand factor.* Biochemistry, 1987. 26(25): p. 8099-109.

[15] Matsui, T., K. Titani, and T. Mizuochi, *Structures of the asparagine-linked oligosaccharide chains of human von Willebrand factor. Occurrence of blood group A, B, and H(O) structures.* J Biol Chem, 1992. 267(13): p. 8723-31.

[16] Voorberg, J., et al., *Assembly and routing of von Willebrand factor variants: the requirements for disulfide-linked dimerization reside within the carboxy-terminal 151 amino acids.* J Cell Biol, 1991. 113(1): p. 195-205.

[17] Sporn, L.A., V.J. Marder, and D.D. Wagner, *Inducible secretion of large, biologically potent von Willebrand factor multimers.* Cell, 1986. 46(2): p. 185-90.

[18] Wagner, D.D., J.B. Olmsted, and V.J. Marder, *Immunolocalization of von Willebrand protein in Weibel-Palade bodies of human endothelial cells.* J Cell Biol, 1982. 95(1): p. 355-60.

[19] Cramer, E.M., et al., *Eccentric localization of von Willebrand factor in an internal structure of platelet alpha-granule resembling that of Weibel-Palade bodies.* Blood, 1985. 66(3): p. 710-3.

[20] Ruggeri, Z.M. and T.S. Zimmerman, *The complex multimeric composition of factor VIII/von Willebrand factor.* Blood, 1981. 57(6): p. 1140-3.

[21] Tsai, H.M., et al., *Multimeric composition of endothelial cell-derived von Willebrand factor.* Blood, 1989. 73(8): p. 2074-6.

[22] Padilla, A., et al., *P-selectin anchors newly released ultralarge von Willebrand factor multimers to the endothelial cell surface.* Blood, 2004. 103(6): p. 2150-6.

[23] Fujikawa, K., et al., *Purification of human von Willebrand factor-cleaving protease and its identification as a new member of the metalloproteinase family.* Blood, 2001. 98(6): p. 1662-6.

[24] Gerritsen, H.E., et al., *Partial amino acid sequence of purified von Willebrand factor-cleaving protease.* Blood, 2001. 98(6): p. 1654-61.

[25] Levy, G.G., et al., *Mutations in a member of the ADAMTS gene family cause thrombotic thrombocytopenic purpura.* Nature, 2001. 413(6855): p. 488-94.

[26] Soejima, K., et al., *A novel human metalloprotease synthesized in the liver and secreted into the blood: possibly, the von Willebrand factor-cleaving protease?* J Biochem, 2001. 130(4): p. 475-80.

[27] Zheng, X., et al., *Structure of von Willebrand factor-cleaving protease (ADAMTS-13), a metalloprotease involved in thrombotic thrombocytopenic purpura.* J Biol Chem, 2001. 276(44): p. 41059-63.

[28] Dobrkovska, A., U. Krzensk, and J.R. Chediak, *Pharmacokinetics, efficacy and safety of Humate-P in von Willebrand disease.* Haemophilia, 1998. 4 Suppl 3: p. 33-9.

[29] Menache, D., et al., *Pharmacokinetics of von Willebrand factor and factor VIIIC in patients with severe von Willebrand disease (type 3 VWD): estimation of the rate of factor VIIIC synthesis. Cooperative Study Groups.* Br J Haematol, 1996. 94(4): p. 740-5.

[30] Lenting, P.J., et al., *An experimental model to study the in vivo survival of von Willebrand factor. Basic aspects and application to the R1205H mutation.* J Biol Chem, 2004. 279(13): p. 12102-9.

[31] Tsai, H.M., *Physiologic cleavage of von Willebrand factor by a plasma protease is dependent on its conformation and requires calcium ion.* Blood, 1996. 87(10): p. 4235-44.

[32] Furlan, M., et al., *von Willebrand factor-cleaving protease in thrombotic thrombocytopenic purpura and the hemolytic-uremic syndrome.* N Engl J Med, 1998. 339(22): p. 1578-84.

[33] Moake, J.L., et al., *Unusually large plasma factor VIII:von Willebrand factor multimers in chronic relapsing thrombotic thrombocytopenic purpura.* N Engl J Med, 1982. 307(23): p. 1432-5.

[34] Tsai, H.M. and E.C. Lian, *Antibodies to von Willebrand factor-cleaving protease in acute thrombotic thrombocytopenic purpura.* N Engl J Med, 1998. 339(22): p. 1585-94.

[35] Hulstein, J.J., et al., *A novel nanobody that detects the gain-of-function phenotype of von Willebrand factor in ADAMTS-13 deficiency and von Willebrand disease type 2B.* Blood, 2005. 106(9): p. 3035-42.

[36] Siedlecki, C.A., et al., *Shear-dependent changes in the three-dimensional structure of human von Willebrand factor.* Blood, 1996. 88(8): p. 2939-50.

[37] Schneider, S.W., et al., *Shear-induced unfolding triggers adhesion of von Willebrand factor fibers.* Proc Natl Acad Sci U S A, 2007. 104(19): p. 7899-903.

[38] Di Stasio, E. and R. De Cristofaro, *The effect of shear stress on protein conformation: Physical forces operating on biochemical systems: The case of von Willebrand factor.* Biophys Chem, 2010. 153(1): p. 1-8.

[39] Di Stasio, E., et al., *Kinetic study of von Willebrand factor self-aggregation induced by ristocetin.* Biophys Chem, 2009. 144(3): p. 101-7.

[40] Hartleib, J., et al., *Protein A is the von Willebrand factor binding protein on Staphylococcus aureus.* Blood, 2000. 96(6): p. 2149-56.

[41] Petri, B., et al., *von Willebrand factor promotes leukocyte extravasation.* Blood, 2010. 116(22): p. 4712-9.

[42] Starke, R.D., et al., *Endothelial von Willebrand factor regulates angiogenesis.* Blood, 2011. 117(3): p. 1071-80.
[43] Fressinaud, E. and D. Meyer, *International survey of patients with von Willebrand disease and angiodysplasia.* Thromb Haemost, 1993. 70(3): p. 546.
[44] Marchese, M., et al., *Duodenal and gastric Dieulafoy's lesions in a patient with type 2A von Willebrand's disease.* Gastrointest Endosc, 2005. 61(2): p. 322-5.
[45] Moschcowitz, E., *An acute febrile pleiochromic anemia with hyaline thrombosis of the terminal arterioles and capillaries: an undescribed disease. 1925.* Mt Sinai J Med, 2003. 70(5): p. 352-5.
[46] Kiss, J.E., *Thrombotic thrombocytopenic purpura: recognition and management.* Int J Hematol, 2010. 91(1): p. 36-45.
[47] Tsai, H.M., *Pathophysiology of thrombotic thrombocytopenic purpura.* Int J Hematol, 2010. 91(1): p. 1-19.
[48] Amorosi, E.L. and J.E. Ultmann, *Thrombotic thrombocytopenic purpura: report of 16 cases and review of the literature.* Medicine (Baltimore), 1966. 45: p. 139-159.
[49] Cohen, J.A., M.E. Brecher, and N. Bandarenko, *Cellular source of serum lactate dehydrogenase elevation in patients with thrombotic thrombocytopenic purpura.* J Clin Apher, 1998. 13(1): p. 16-9.
[50] Verbeke, L., M. Delforge, and D. Dierickx, *Current insight into thrombotic thrombocytopenic purpura.* Blood Coagul Fibrinolysis, 2010. 21(1): p. 3-10.
[51] Zhou, Z., et al., *Von Willebrand factor, ADAMTS-13, and thrombotic thrombocytopenic purpura.* Semin Thromb Hemost, 2010. 36(1): p. 71-81.
[52] Ferrari, S., et al., *IgG subclass distribution of anti-ADAMTS-13 antibodies in patients with acquired thrombotic thrombocytopenic purpura.* J Thromb Haemost, 2009. 7(10): p. 1703-10.
[53] Moake, J., et al., *Solvent/detergent-treated plasma suppresses shear-induced platelet aggregation and prevents episodes of thrombotic thrombocytopenic purpura.* Blood, 1994. 84(2): p. 490-7.
[54] Rock, G.A., et al., *Comparison of plasma exchange with plasma infusion in the treatment of thrombotic thrombocytopenic purpura. Canadian Apheresis Study Group.* N Engl J Med, 1991. 325(6): p. 393-7.
[55] Shumak, K.H., G.A. Rock, and R.C. Nair, *Late relapses in patients successfully treated for thrombotic thrombocytopenic purpura. Canadian Apheresis Group.* Ann Intern Med, 1995. 122(8): p. 569-72.
[56] Kremer Hovinga, J.A. and S.C. Meyer, *Current management of thrombotic thrombocytopenic purpura.* Curr Opin Hematol, 2008. 15(5): p. 445-50.
[57] Blake-Haskins, J.A., R.J. Lechleider, and R.J. Kreitman, *Thrombotic microangiopathy with targeted cancer agents.* Clin Cancer Res, 2011. 17(18): p. 5858-66.
[58] Caramazza, D., et al., *Relapsing or refractory idiopathic thrombotic thrombocytopenic purpura-hemolytic uremic syndrome: the role of rituximab.* Transfusion, 2010. 50(12): p. 2753-60.
[59] Noris, P. and C.L. Balduini, *Investigational drugs in thrombotic thrombocytopenic purpura.* Expert Opin Investig Drugs, 2011. 20(8): p. 1087-98.
[60] Scully, M., et al., *A phase 2 study of the safety and efficacy of rituximab with plasma exchange in acute acquired thrombotic thrombocytopenic purpura.* Blood, 2011. 118(7): p. 1746-53.

[61] Kiss, J.E. *Major Clinical Trials in Apheresis: TTP.* in *American Society For Apheresis (ASFA).* 2010. New Orleans.

[62] Gasser, C., et al., *[Hemolytic-uremic syndrome: bilateral necrosis of the renal cortex in acute acquired hemolytic anemia].* Schweiz Med Wochenschr, 1955. 85(38-39): p. 905-9.

[63] Moake, J.L., *Haemolytic-uraemic syndrome: basic science.* Lancet, 1994. 343(8894): p. 393-7.

[64] Obrig, T.G., *Pathogenesis of Shiga toxin (verotoxin)-induced endothelial cell injury* Hemolytic uremic syndrome and thrombotic thrombocytopenic purpura. , ed. B.S. Kaplan, R.S. Trompeter, and J.L. Moake. 1992, New York: Marcel Dekker. 405-19.

[65] Ray, P.E. and X.H. Liu, *Pathogenesis of Shiga toxin-induced hemolytic uremic syndrome.* Pediatr Nephrol, 2001. 16(10): p. 823-39.

[66] Bell, W.R., et al., *Improved survival in thrombotic thrombocytopenic purpura-hemolytic uremic syndrome. Clinical experience in 108 patients.* N Engl J Med, 1991. 325(6): p. 398-403.

[67] Karmali, M.A., et al., *The association between idiopathic hemolytic uremic syndrome and infection by verotoxin-producing Escherichia coli.* J Infect Dis, 1985. 151(5): p. 775-82.

[68] Gutterman, L.A. and T.D. Stevenson, *Treatment of thrombotic thrombocytopenic purpura with vincristine.* Jama, 1982. 247(10): p. 1433-6.

[69] Bennett, C.L., et al., *Thrombotic thrombocytopenic purpura associated with clopidogrel.* N Engl J Med, 2000. 342(24): p. 1773-7.

[70] Bennett, C.L., et al., *Thrombotic thrombocytopenic purpura associated with ticlopidine. A review of 60 cases.* Ann Intern Med, 1998. 128(7): p. 541-4.

[71] Rosove, M.H., W.G. Ho, and D. Goldfinger, *Ineffectiveness of aspirin and dipyridamole in the treatment of thrombotic thrombocytopenic purpura.* Ann Intern Med, 1982. 96(1): p. 27-33.

[72] Tsai, H.M., et al., *Antibody inhibitors to von Willebrand factor metalloproteinase and increased binding of von Willebrand factor to platelets in ticlopidine-associated thrombotic thrombocytopenic purpura.* Ann Intern Med, 2000. 132(10): p. 794-9.

[73] Saito, I., et al., *Nontraditional risk factors for coronary heart disease incidence among persons with diabetes: the Atherosclerosis Risk in Communities (ARIC) Study.* Ann Intern Med, 2000. 133(2): p. 81-91.

[74] Spiel, A.O., J.C. Gilbert, and B. Jilma, *von Willebrand factor in cardiovascular disease: focus on acute coronary syndromes.* Circulation, 2008. 117(11): p. 1449-59.

[75] Frankel, D.S., et al., *Von Willebrand factor, type 2 diabetes mellitus, and risk of cardiovascular disease: the framingham offspring study.* Circulation, 2008. 118(24): p. 2533-9.

[76] Hanson, E., et al., *Plasma levels of von Willebrand factor in the etiologic subtypes of ischemic stroke.* J Thromb Haemost, 2011. 9(2): p. 275-81.

[77] Wieberdink, R.G., et al., *High von Willebrand factor levels increase the risk of stroke: the Rotterdam study.* Stroke, 2010. 41(10): p. 2151-6.

[78] Hund-Georgiadis, M., et al., *Characterization of cerebral microangiopathy using 3 Tesla MRI: correlation with neurological impairment and vascular risk factors.* J Magn Reson Imaging, 2002. 15(1): p. 1-7.

[79] Scarpelli, M., et al., *MRI and pathological examination of post-mortem brains: the problem of white matter high signal areas.* Neuroradiology, 1994. 36(5): p. 393-8.

[80] Froissart, A., et al., *Efficacy and safety of first-line rituximab in severe, acquired thrombotic thrombocytopenic purpura with a suboptimal response to plasma exchange. Experience of the French Thrombotic Microangiopathies Reference Center.* Crit Care Med, 2011.